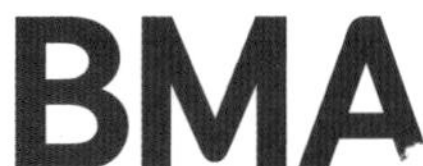

Managing Hot Flushes with Group Cognitive Behaviour Therapy

Following the success of *Managing Hot Flushes and Night Sweats* which outlines a self-help, CBT-based programme for dealing with menopausal symptoms, Myra Hunter and Melanie Smith have developed a pioneering group treatment for women going through the menopause. *Managing Hot Flushes with Group Cognitive Behaviour Therapy* is an evidence-based manual drawing on their research which has demonstrated, in randomised controlled trials, that Group CBT effectively reduces the impact of hot flushes and night sweats. The treatment is effective for women going through a natural menopause and for women who have menopausal symptoms following breast cancer treatments and for other groups of women who have troublesome symptoms. This manual provides health professionals with everything they need to run groups to help women to manage hot flushes and night sweats.

Managing Hot Flushes with Group Cognitive Behaviour Therapy equips health professionals with knowledge, skills and materials to run groups to help women to manage menopausal symptoms in six (or four) weekly sessions without the need for medication. It is easy to use with a companion audio exercise and downloadable resources online, as well as PowerPoint slides, homework sheets and diaries. Following Group CBT women have the information, practical skills and strategies to help them to cope with hot flushes and night sweats, and also report improvements in sleep and quality of life. This manual will be an essential resource for nurses, psychologists, counsellors, psychological wellbeing practitioners and cognitive behaviour therapists working in health care and voluntary settings.

Myra Hunter is Professor of Clinical Health Psychology at the Institute of Psychiatry, King's College London. She has worked in the area of women's health for over 30 years and has over 150 publications including six books. Her research on menopause has established her as an international expert in the field.

Melanie Smith is a clinical psychologist, who has specialised in helping people to manage physical health conditions using cognitive behaviour therapy (CBT). She researched and provided the CBT for women with hot flushes in the MENOS trials at King's College London and is currently with Salford Pain Centre, Manchester.

Managing Hot Flushes with Group Cognitive Behaviour Therapy

An evidence-based treatment manual for health professionals

Myra Hunter and Melanie Smith

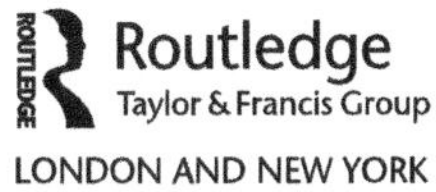

LONDON AND NEW YORK

First published 2015
by Routledge
27 Church Road, Hove, East Sussex, BN3 2FA

and by Routledge
711 Third Avenue, New York, NY 10017

Routledge is an imprint of the Taylor & Francis Group, an informa business

British Library Cataloguing in Publication Data
A catalogue record for this book is available from the British Library

Library of Congress Cataloging in Publication Data
Hunter, Myra, author.
Managing hot flushes with group cognitive behaviour therapy : an evidence based treatment manual for health professionals / Myra Hunter and Melanie Smith.
p. ; cm.
Includes bibliographical references and index.
ISBN 978-1-138-02614-8 (hbk) – ISBN 978-1-138-02615-5 (pbk) –
ISBN 978-1-315-76419-1 (ebk)
I. Smith, Melanie, 1975- , author. II. Title.
[DNLM: 1. Cognitive Therapy–methods. 2. Hot Flashes–therapy.
3. Evidence-Based Medicine. 4. Psychotherapy, Group–methods. WP 580]
RC489.C62
616.89'1425–dc23

2014024381

ISBN: 978-1-138-02614-8 (hbk)
ISBN: 978-1-138-02615-5 (pbk)
ISBN: 978-1-315-76419-1 (ebk)

Typeset in Frutiger
by RefineCatch Limited, Bungay, Suffolk, UK

Printed and bound by CPI Group (UK) Ltd, Croydon, CR0 4YY

Dedication

This book is dedicated to all the women who took part in our research on the treatment of hot flushes and night sweats and who participated in the Group CBT. We learnt such a lot from all of you.

Contents

List of illustrations ix
Foreword xi
Acknowledgements xiii

1 Introduction **1**

2 Session 1: Psycho-education and the cognitive behavioural model **19**

3 Session 2: Stress management, improving wellbeing and identifying precipitants **29**

4 Session 3: Managing hot flushes using a cognitive behavioural approach **43**

5 Session 4: Managing night sweats and improving sleep (part one) **59**

6 Session 5: Managing night sweats and improving sleep (part two) **73**

7 Session 6: Review and maintaining changes **83**

Appendix: Handouts 97
Slides 125
Resources 175
References 183
Index 189

Illustrations

FIGURES

1.1 The thermo-neutral zone (TNZ) and hot flushes 6
1.2 A cognitive behavioural model of hot flushes and night sweats 8
1.3 Hot Flush Rating Scale: frequency and problem-rating 14
1.4 Hot flush daily diary 15
4.1 Sleep diary 57
5.1 Stages of sleep 63
6.1 A continuum of predictions during the night about the next day compared with experience 78

TABLE

1.1 Proposed measures, cognitive and behavioural mechanisms in CBT interventions for hot flushes and night sweats 9

Foreword

Many women go through the menopause without problems. For some, it changes everything. Hot flushes can be a minor embarrassment or a major disruption to sleep and daily life over many years. Yet, these problems are often underestimated, belittled and largely hidden. Medication, such as hormone replacement therapy, can be helpful, but none come without risks or side effects. Furthermore, hormone replacement therapy is not available for women who have had, or are at risk of, breast cancer. The provision of alternative methods of managing menopausal problems is variable, especially as there is little evidence to support the efficacy of these methods.

Myra Hunter has dedicated her career to working in women's health and, with Melanie Smith, has spent many years developing and testing the efficacy of cognitive behaviour therapy (CBT) as an intervention to help women at midlife. They have gained considerable knowledge and expertise in this area, identifying what women find helpful and honing the intervention. They have delivered courses to many groups of women who have benefited from this approach to menopause management and have now pooled this expertise into a manual for other health professionals.

This manual comes with good explanations around menopause and the theory underlying the intervention, as well as comprehensive detail as to how to run the Group CBT intervention and the slides to accompany each session. This is a detailed and excellent resource for any health professional wishing to offer a service to help women with menopausal difficulties.

Dr Deborah Fenlon, Senior Lecturer, University of Southampton
Clinical Advisor for Breast Cancer Care and Chair of the
National Cancer Research Institute Clinical Studies Group
for breast cancer working party on symptom
management (vasomotor).

Acknowledgements

We would like to thank all the women who have taken part in our research studies over the years and especially those who participated in our recent trials and provided such detailed and useful feedback. We are grateful to colleagues who contributed to the research, including Shirley Coventry, Lih-Mei Liao, Beverley Ayers, Eleanor Mann, Janet Balabanovic and Chinea Eziefula, and to Sue Gessler and Kathy Abernethy for their helpful comments. Thank you also to Susannah Frearson and Joanne Forshaw at Routledge for their ongoing support and advice.

Grateful acknowledgement is made to the following for permission to include previously published material:

Figure 1.1 'The thermo-neutral zone (TNZ) and hot flushes' has been adapted and reproduced from Archer et al. (2011), *Climacteric*, with kind permission from Informa Healthcare.

Figure 1.2 'A cognitive behavioural model of hot flushes and night sweats' has been adapted and reproduced from Hunter and Mann (2010), *Journal of Psychosomatic Research*, with kind permission from Elsevier.

Figure 5.1 'Stages of sleep' has been reproduced from Luciddreamexplorers (http://ygraph.com/chart/2076). Permission to use the chart is granted by Bulb media on the condition that it is linked back to: http://www.LucidDreamExplorers.com/dreamscience/

Handout 3 'Hot flushes and night sweats: relationships between physical changes, thoughts, mood, behaviour and lifestyle' has been adapted and reproduced from Hunter (2003), *Journal of Reproductive and Infant Psychology*, with kind permission from Taylor & Francis.

Handout 10 'Survey results: What do other people think about hot flushes?' has been adapted and reproduced from Smith et al. (2011), *Maturitas*, with kind permission from Elsevier.

Note

Throughout the book any names of women have been changed to preserve their privacy.

1

Introduction

This is a treatment manual for a Group cognitive behaviour therapy (Group CBT) programme to help women to manage menopausal hot flushes and night sweats. The following chapters outline the Group CBT in detail. The treatment is designed for women who have menopausal symptoms and who are having a 'natural' menopause, as well as for women who have had a menopause following surgery or medical treatment. We include guidance for women who have symptoms following treatments for breast cancer which can induce or exacerbate the symptoms, and for whom medical treatments, such as hormone replacement therapy (HRT), may not be recommended. The Group CBT is also appropriate for women who have menopause at a younger age, i.e. before 40 years, or premature menopause, as well as during midlife.

The manual is best used in conjunction with a practical skills-based training course, and while it has been developed by clinical psychologists it is designed to be implemented by health professionals, such as clinical nurse specialists and primary care staff, who have had some training and who can access clinical supervision. The manual includes cognitive behaviour therapy skills, so some knowledge and experience of this approach would be advantageous.

The Group CBT is psycho-educational and evidence-based, so in the following sections we provide information about the menopause, hot flushes and the research carried out to develop and to evaluate the treatment. Following this, practical aspects of assessment and preparation for Group CBT are described.

THE MENOPAUSE

Definitions

The menopause occurs on average between the ages of 50 and 51, in most Western cultures, and specifically refers to a woman's last menstrual period. The menopause is a fairly universal experience for women if they live long enough, although for some the process of the menopause is influenced by surgery or disease. However, the last menstrual period takes place within a gradual process involving physiological changes as well as age and psychosocial changes, and within varied cultural contexts (Hunter and Rendall 2007).

The definition of the menopause that has been widely used is based on that of the World Health Organization (Sherman 2005; World Health Organization 1981), which refers to the menopause as the 'permanent cessation of menstruation resulting from loss of ovarian follicular activity'. The following stages of the menopause transition are based on menstrual patterns:

- Premenopause is defined by regular menstruation.
- Perimenopause includes the phase immediately prior to the menopause and the first year after menopause and is defined by changes in the regularity of menstruation during the previous 12 months.
- Postmenopausal women who have not menstruated during the past 12 months.

Some women who have had surgery, such as a hysterectomy (removal of the womb) or oophorectomy (removal of the ovaries), or those who are taking hormone therapy (HT) may be difficult to classify. Interestingly, the classification of postmenopause can only be made in retrospect because it is impossible to know which menstrual period will be the last. More recently, the Stages of Reproductive Ageing Workshop (STRAW) created a system, which more accurately describes reproductive status in healthy women (Harlow et al. 2012) (see STRAW definitions box below). Parallel changes in menstruation, hormonal changes and experience of hot flushes and night sweats across women's lifespans are included.

Stages of Reproductive Ageing Workshop (STRAW) definitions:

- Reproductive stage: includes menarche (onset of menstrual periods) with variable menstruation initially; it can take several years for regular menstrual cycles to develop, which are typically every 21–35 days. Across this phase, which usually lasts from adolescence to late 40s, fairly regular menstruation continues, but there can be some changes in flow (sometimes becoming heavy) and changes in length of the cycle.
- Menopause transition: includes early transition (regular menstruation but changes in menstrual cycle length), and late menopause transition (two or more missed menstrual periods and at least one interval of 60 days or more between menstrual periods), which happens one to three years before the final menstrual period. During this stage follicle stimulating hormone (FSH) levels tend to rise (this hormone is working hard to try to produce ovulation) and oestrogen levels start to reduce. Hot flushes are likely to occur during the late menopause transition.
- Menopause: the last menstrual period (LMP).
- Postmenopause: this stage is divided into early (up to six years after the LMP) and late (the subsequent years). Early postmenopause is characterised by hormonal changes and hot flushes, which tend to stabilise during the late postmenopause.

Additional terms, such as 'climacteric syndrome' and 'menopause syndrome' have been used to refer to a host of physical and emotional experiences that may or may not be related to hormone or menstrual changes, including hot flushes, vaginal dryness, loss of libido, depression, anxiety, irritability, poor memory, loss of concentration, mood swings, insomnia, tiredness, aching limbs, loss of energy and dry skin. Similarly, 'the change', 'change of life' and 'midlife crisis' are terms of use that reflect the view that the menopause is associated with general psychological and social adaptations of midlife. In terms of timing, midlife often coincides with changes in personal and social relationships and sometimes with life events such as illness, death of parents, dealing with adolescent children and children leaving home, as well as perceived personal and social consequences of reaching the age of 50. But this is certainly not the case for all women, and, if changes do happen, their impact and whether they are attributed to the menopause or not will be influenced by the social, economic and cultural context in which women live.

Nevertheless, the menopause has for centuries been associated with emotional and physical problems, particularly in Western cultures, and negative assumptions about its impact upon sexual function, femininity, ageing and women's mental health are still prevalent in the media today. In contrast, studies of menopause across cultures suggest wide variations in the perception and experience of physical changes and the meanings of the menopause. Women living in North America and Europe tend to report more hot flushes than those living in China, Japan and the Indian subcontinent (Freeman and Sherif 2007). Higher prevalence rates have also been reported amongst Caucasians, African-Americans and Hispanics compared with Chinese- and Japanese-Americans in a study of women from different ethnic groups living in the USA (Gold et al. 2006). Explanations of these differences include lifestyle (diet, exercise, social factors, and reproductive patterns), which can affect biological processes, as well as beliefs and attitudes to the menopause and the social status of mid-aged and older women (Gupta et al. 2006a; Lock 2005; Melby et al. 2005). There are also qualitative studies that show that women themselves challenge the idea of the menopause as a universally negative phenomenon (Hunter and O'Dea 1997; Hvas 2006). Overall, the menopause can be seen as a bio-psycho-socio-cultural process, the experience of which tends to vary considerably between women and within and between cultures (Archer et al. 2011; Hunter and Rendall 2007). For the majority of women the menopause is seen as a 'normal life-stage' but, at the same time, approximately a quarter of women have troublesome hot flushes and night sweats, that impact on quality of life and for which they seek help.

In the following sections biological and psychosocial aspects of menopause are described, and then the main sections of the chapter focus on hot flushes and the cognitive behavioural approach.

Biological changes

The function of the ovaries and hormone secretion is regulated by the hypothalamo–pituitary–ovarian axis. The main factor influencing the transition from regular menstruation (premenopause) to the perimenopause appears to be the number of ovarian follicles that women have. While at birth there are approximately 700,000 follicles in a woman's ovaries the numbers reduce considerably in the years leading up to the menopause and at the time of the last menstrual period few follicles remain. Follicle stimulating hormone (FSH) concentrations gradually increase in the years leading up to the perimenopause and level of oestradiol gradually reduces.

During the reproductive years oestradiol is the main type of oestrogen that is produced, but after the menopause oestrogen production does not stop because another oestrogen, oestrone, is produced from three main sources: the adrenal cortex, indirectly from the body's fat cells which convert androstenedione to oestrone, and from the ovaries which continue to produce small quantities of androgens which are converted to oestrogens. Testosterone levels stay at approximately the same level after the menopause, being produced by the adrenal glands and by conversion of other hormones (Richardson 1993; Burger 2006).

Psychosocial issues

The menopause is generally viewed as a time of poor emotional and physical health in Western societies and attitudes to the menopause are influenced by historical and cultural beliefs about older women (Flint 1975; Wilbush 1979). Much of the early research was based on clinic samples of women who had actively sought treatment for health problems. Women attending menopause clinics understandably tend to have more health problems, life stresses and low mood than those who do not, as well as differing beliefs about the menopause, such as seeing it as more akin to a disease (Hunter et al. 1997; Guthrie et al. 2003).

Determining the precise relationship between menopause and mood has been a difficult area to research because of numerous methodological issues (defining menopausal stages, measurement of mood and confounding factors of age and social changes). Longitudinal studies have been designed that follow the same women through the menopause transition (Dennerstein et al. 2004; Mishra and Kuh 2012). The main findings from these studies suggest that the menopause is not necessarily associated with psychological symptoms for the majority of healthy women. Therefore, depressed mood should not be attributed automatically to the menopause transition nor expected to occur. Instead, all aspects of a woman's life that might contribute to depression should be considered. Moreover, neutral or positive consequences are also reported. For example, in studies that describe women's accounts of menopause, both positive beliefs and experiences, such as relief from cessation of menstrual periods and risk of pregnancy, tend to be reported, as well as concerns about ageing and negative images of the menopause (Hunter and O'Dea 1997; Perz and Ussher 2008). However, some women do experience mood changes during the perimenopause or transition to menopause, but it is estimated that these represent a relatively small proportion of women in general – about 9–10 per cent – and the evidence suggests that for these women mood tends to return to normal after the menopause (Mishra and Kuh 2012). Factors found to be associated with depressed mood during the menopause transition include: past psychological problems, social difficulties, educational and occupational status, poor health, stressful life events, attitudes to menopause and ageing and early life circumstances and experiences, so these factors also need to be considered (Dennerstein et al. 2004; Woods et al. 2006; Gold et al. 2000; Ayers et al. 2010). In addition, women who have had a surgical menopause and those who have chronic and troublesome hot flushes and night sweats also tend to report more psychological symptoms. Problematic hot flushes and low mood and/or anxiety often occur together and are likely to interact, leading to a vicious cycle. However, overall, the experience of psychosocial factors has been found to have a much stronger association with psychological symptoms than stage of menopause.

With respect to sexual functioning, vaginal dryness is associated with the lower oestrogen levels and occurs more frequently in the postmenopause. In general sexual interest tends to reduce with age and across the menopause transition and is associated with a number of factors including sexual functioning before the menopause, stress, ill health, having problematic night sweats, low mood, relationship status (being in a relationship or having a new partner) and partner's sexual functioning, attitudes towards sex and ageing, as well as cultural background (including beliefs about the importance of sex) (Avis et al. 2005; Dennerstein et al. 2005). There are considerable differences between women in their expectations and experiences of sexual functioning. There is not much research on lesbian women, but there is some evidence from one study that lesbian women with active and fulfilling sex lives tended to communicate openly and were willing to change their sexual repertoire if needed to adapt to menopausal changes (Winterich 2003). There is also some evidence that despite changes in some aspects of sexual functioning with age and menopause, the majority of women who are in relationships report being satisfied and often make adjustments in response to their circumstances, such as ill health, and maintain intimacy in their relationships (Ussher et al. 2013).

MENOPAUSAL SYMPTOMS: HOT FLUSHES AND NIGHT SWEATS

Hot flushes and night sweats, also called vasomotor symptoms, are the main physical signs of menopause, as well as menstrual cycle changes. They are reported by 70–80 per cent of women in Western cultures during the menopause transition (Freeman and Sherif 2007; Andrikoula and Prevelic 2009; Archer et al. 2011), and are commonly described as sensations of heat in the face, neck and chest, frequently accompanied by perspiration and/or shivering. In general, reports of hot flushes increase as women progress from early to the late menopause transition and later gradually reduce. On average, they last for approximately four to five years but there is again wide variation, and recent studies have found that some women continue to have them for over 10 years (Col et al. 2009; Hunter et al. 2011; Freeman et al. 2014).

Although hot flushes are part of normal development given their prevalence, they are problematic for some women; it is estimated that approximately 20–25 per cent of menopausal women seek help for troublesome hot flushes and/or night sweats and they are associated with reduced quality of life (Utian 2005; Ayers and Hunter 2013). While the prevalence rates of night sweats are lower, they are often more distressing than hot flushes because of their association with reduced sleep quality. Sleep disruption is reported by about a quarter of menopausal women and is more common in women who experience frequent night sweats. There is marked variation in the duration, severity, and frequency of hot flushes. Women of low socio-economic status and education, and those who have higher body mass index (BMI), are cigarette smokers and have low levels of physical activity and higher levels of anxiety are more at risk of having troublesome hot flushes (Andrikoula and Prevelic 2009; Sievert et al. 2006; Ford 2004; Thurston et al. 2008; Thurston et al. 2009). However, it is extremely difficult to predict who will have troublesome hot flushes in an individual case.

Hot flushes are also common amongst breast cancer survivors, and tend to be more severe for these women, being associated with sleep problems and reduced health-related quality of life (Gupta et al. 2006b; Hunter et al. 2004; Fenlon and Rogers 2007; Morgan et al. 2014). They can be induced or exacerbated by treatments such as chemotherapy and by endocrine therapies, for example Tamoxifen (Howell et al. 2005). In addition, women taking hormone replacement therapy (HRT) are generally advised to stop the treatment because HRT might increase risk of cancer recurrence. Menopausal symptoms tend to occur after a period of intensive treatment and at a time when women are working to get their lives back to normal and have less contact with their clinical teams. For some women the experience of treatment-related hot flushes has a negative impact on their adherence to endocrine treatments, which are used to reduce risk of recurrence, such as Tamoxifen (Hershman et al. 2011). For younger women the experience of the abrupt onset of menopausal symptoms can be particularly distressing because of concerns about fertility, as well as the psychological and physical impact of being 'menopausal' at a young age (Thewes et al. 2004).

Therefore, there is a need for safe and effective treatment options for (i) women who do not want to take medical treatments for hot flushes, or for (ii) women who have flushes following breast cancer treatment, for whom non-hormonal treatments, such as cognitive behaviour therapy, are often preferred (Hunter et al. 2004).

Physiology: The exact cause of hot flushes and night sweats is unknown, but they appear to be associated with the rate of change of plasma oestrogen, rather than levels of oestrogen, which influences the thermoregulatory system via the hypothalamus (Freedman 2005; Archer et al. 2011). Hence hot flushes are more prevalent following rapid withdrawal of oestrogen, for example, following surgical menopause or adjuvant chemotherapy for breast cancer. As a result of oestrogen withdrawal the hypothalamic set point temperature is altered and autonomic reactions to cool down are more easily activated. This results in flushing and sweating of the skin by peripheral vasodilation. Freedman (2005) proposes that there is a narrowed thermoneutral zone (TNZ) in women who have hot flushes resulting in hot flushes being triggered by small elevations in core body temperature, caused by changes in ambient temperature or other internal or external triggers, such as anxiety, coffee or alcohol. This physiological model provides a framework with which to understand the role of psychological factors and psychological interventions for hot flushes (see Figure 1.1).

Anxiety is associated with elevated levels of norepinephrine, a neurotransmitter that is known to play a role in thermoregulation. Stress also produces increased sympathetic responses, increasing norepinephrine and serotonin, which may affect the TNZ in women with hot flushes. There is evidence from a laboratory study (Swartzman et al. 1990) that stress potentiates hot flushes by lowering the hot flush threshold in the hypothalamus, so that hot flushes are more likely to occur if women are generally stressed. However, triggers or precipitants of hot flushes have also been identified. Approximately 50 per cent of flushes can be triggered by internal and external events, such as hot drinks, changes in ambient temperature, rushing, stress or eating hot or spicy foods (Hunter and Liao 1995; Gannon et al. 1987).

Experience of hot flushes: Studies of women's subjective reports of hot flushes have found that the experience is broadly similar among well women and breast cancer survivors (Carpenter et al. 2002); although in general hot flushes are reported as being more severe by women who have had breast cancer treatments, and specific meanings have been found to be relevant to women following breast cancer treatment, such as flushes being a reminder of one's body feeling out of control (Fenlon and Rogers 2007).

Subjective experience includes reported frequency, the extent to which they are problematic, as well as cognitive appraisals (thoughts and beliefs) and emotional and behavioural reactions to them (Hunter and Mann 2010). We have examined cognitive

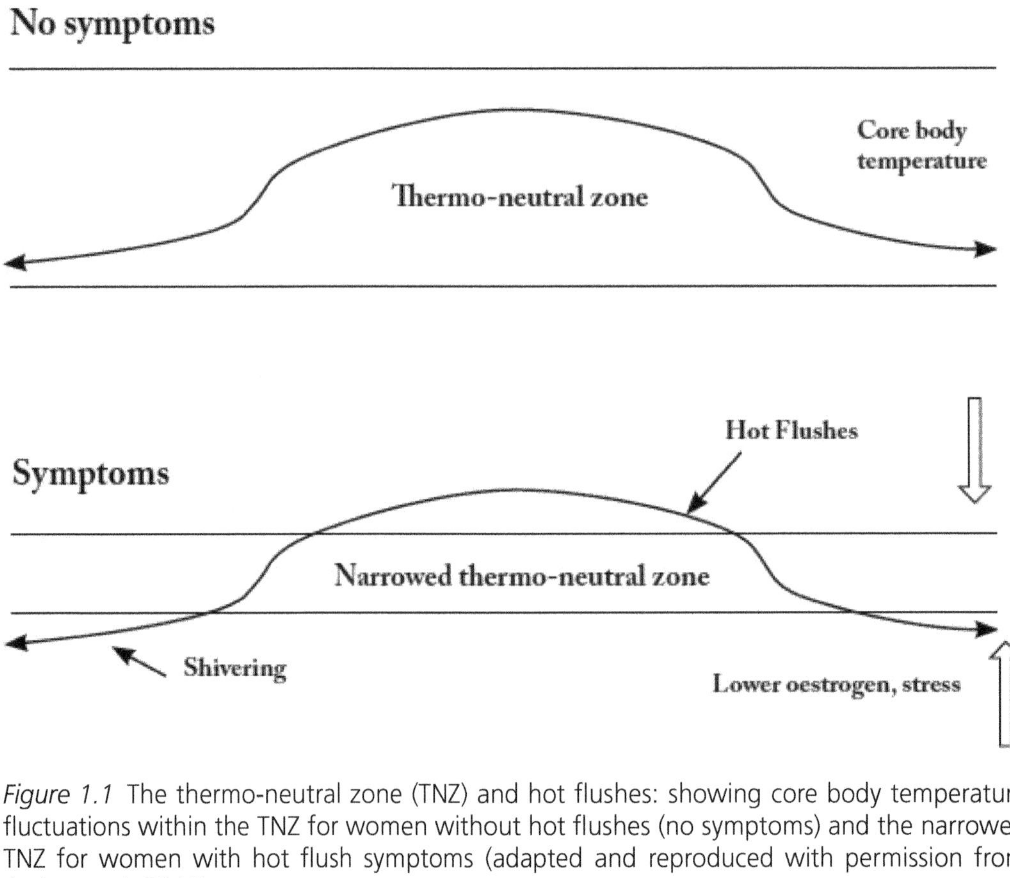

Figure 1.1 The thermo-neutral zone (TNZ) and hot flushes: showing core body temperature fluctuations within the TNZ for women without hot flushes (no symptoms) and the narrowed TNZ for women with hot flush symptoms (adapted and reproduced with permission from Archer et al. 2011)

and behavioural responses in well women (Rendall et al. 2008; Hunter et al. 2011) and breast cancer patients (Hunter et al. 2009b). We found that certain cognitions (thoughts), emotions, and behaviours are commonly reported by the women who have troublesome hot flushes and night sweats:

1. Cognitions: automatic thoughts and beliefs that other people will have negative thoughts about them (that they are unattractive, stupid, old etc.) if they have flushes in social situations; thoughts that hot flushes are uncontrollable and overwhelming; unhelpful beliefs about night sweats and sleep (that they will never get back to sleep, and that they will feel terrible the next day).
2. Emotions: embarrassment, anxiety, worrying and frustration.
3. Behaviours: attempts to cool down, avoidance of activities and situations, problems in communication with others.

The theme 'social anxiety/embarrassment' was the most commonly mentioned, particularly when women had flushes at work or in public places. Women often describe negative beliefs about themselves when having flushes in social situations and believe that other people think that they are stupid or unattractive, or old and 'past it' (Smith et al. 2011). These thoughts or cognitions are similar to those of people with social anxiety, in that there is concern about behaving in a way that will be humiliating or embarrassing, but there is less intense anxiety and fear of having panic attacks or fainting. Some of the behavioural strategies mentioned, such as avoidance of social situations and use of preventative or cooling behaviours (such as covering the face and carrying fans, wipes etc.), are similar to those that have been shown to be maintaining behaviours in social anxiety. Avoidance and preventative behaviours may reduce the opportunities for the development of alternative more neutral interpretations. Catastrophic thoughts such as, 'I cannot possibly concentrate', 'It is terrible and I feel that it is never going to get any better' tend to be associated with greater distress (Reynolds 1999; 2000).

There are also elements of shame and stigma in the women's responses in social situations. Women describe feeling that a private event (menopause) is being publically disclosed when they have hot flushes, because they are observable. It could be argued that they were reacting to negative social meanings of menopause, for example menopause has been linked to ageing, loss of femininity and value and even with insanity (Hunter and O'Dea 1997). The strategy of communicating with openness and humour is likely to be helpful in countering negative social assumptions, and might help to reduce social anxiety and improve mood.

Another set of cognitions is related to beliefs about control – that the flushes were overwhelming, might never end and couldn't be controlled. An alternative strategy mentioned by the women is to accept that they are happening and to try to carry on with what they are doing, which is consistent with newer therapeutic approaches such as mindfulness (Kabat-Zinn 2003; Carmody et al. 2011) and acceptance and commitment therapy (Hayes et al. 2004).

Research on sleep and insomnia suggests that negative cognitions, such as 'I'll never get back to sleep' and 'If I wake up at night I'll feel terrible the next day', are associated with maintenance of sleep problems and tiredness. These cognitions increase anxiety and arousal, which leads to increased wakefulness and can result in daytime fatigue (Harvey 2002). Strategies such as automatically getting up, cooling down and going back to bed with neutral thoughts and acceptance are likely to be helpful, as are not taking daytime naps and following general advice about 'sleep hygiene' (Espie 2006). Cognitive behavioural approaches to sleep problems have been found to be effective in mid aged and older populations (Irwin et al. 2006).

A COGNITIVE BEHAVIOURAL MODEL OF HOT FLUSHES

We have developed a cognitive behavioural model of hot flushes, which describes possible relationships between biological, cognitive, behavioural and environmental factors influencing hot flushes, and outlines the possible mechanisms by which cognitive behavioural intervention components are hypothesised to impact on hot flushes (Hunter and Mann 2010). The Group CBT contained in this manual is based on this cognitive behavioural model (see Figure 1.2).

The model draws upon theories of symptom perception (Cioffi 1991; Pennebaker 1982), self-regulation theory (Leventhal et al. 1984) and cognitive behavioural models (Hunter 2003). There are four main sections:

1. Information input,
2. Detection and attribution,
3. Cognitive appraisal, and
4. Behaviour.

Information input refers to the relationship between oestrogen reduction and central thermoregulation. The detection and attribution section describes how the physiological events may then be perceived or identified as hot flushes. Cognitive appraisal includes the interpretation or meaning of the flushes, for example whether they are evaluated as problematic or bothersome. Finally the behaviour section refers to help seeking or other behavioural strategies, which may ameliorate or exacerbate

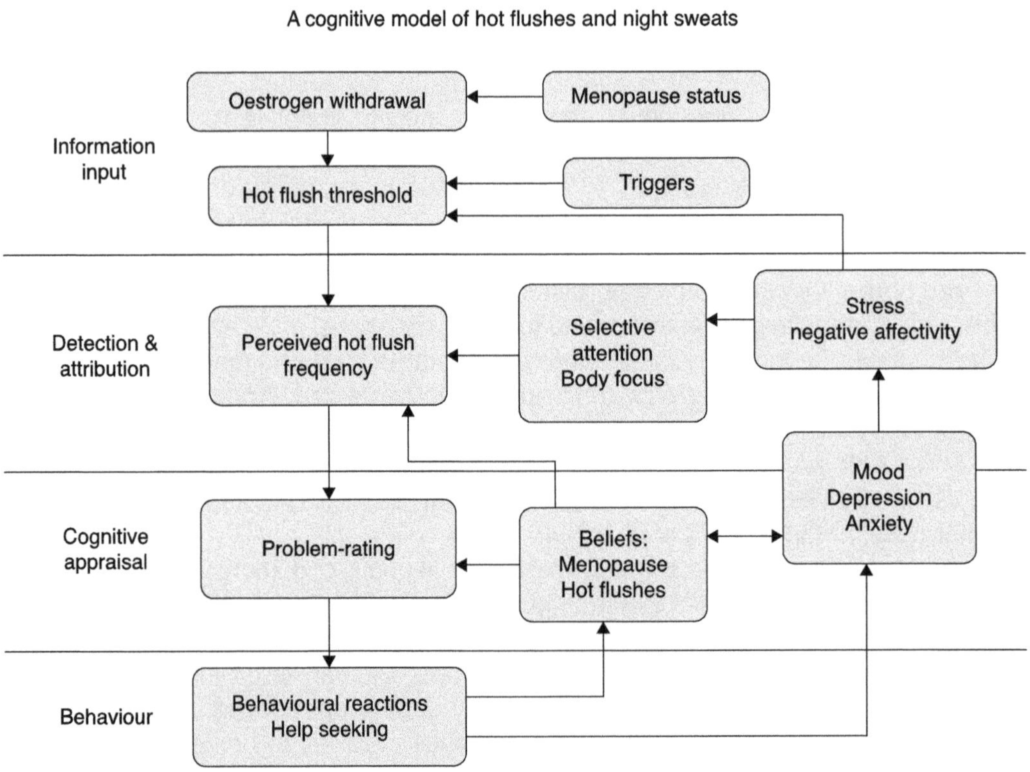

Figure 1.2 A cognitive behavioural model of hot flushes and night sweats (adapted and reproduced with permission from Hunter and Mann 2010)

hot flushes. The model applies to symptomatic menopausal women, i.e. women with hot flushes, and is described in detail in Hunter and Mann (2010). The model provides a framework that can be used to understand the ways in which psychological treatments might work; these are used in the Group CBT and are outlined in Table 1.1.

We have tested this model in a recent study of 140 women with hot flushes, who were measured both subjectively and physiologically. We found that stress, anxiety and bodily focus of attention (somatic amplification) predicted hot flush problem-rating (how troublesome the symptoms were) but that they had this effect mainly through their impact on hot flush beliefs or cognitions (Hunter and Chilcot 2013); hot flush frequency, smoking and alcohol intake also predicted hot flush problem-rating. Hot flush beliefs and behaviours were associated with one other (particularly social anxieties and avoidance, and beliefs about coping and control and unhelpful behaviours) and predicted how problematic hot flushes were experienced. These results support the cognitive behavioural model, in that psychological factors impact upon symptom perception and cognitive appraisal of hot flushes.

Table 1.1 Proposed measures, cognitive and behavioural mechanisms in CBT interventions for hot flushes and night sweats

Stage of Model of HF/NS	*Measures*	*Mechanism*	*Intervention component*
Information input	Hot flush frequency assessed by sternal skin conductance or other physiological measures	Raise physiological HF threshold Reduce triggers	Paced breathing Stress management Monitor and modify triggers
Symptom perception	Self-reported hot flush frequency Stress Negative affectivity Somatic amplification	Shift attentional focus Improve mood Increase accurate attribution of sensations	Paced breathing Stress management Cognitive therapy Provide information about aetiology, causes and impacts of HF/NS and menopause
Cognitive appraisal	Hot flush problem-rating HF belief scale Menopause representations questionnaire (MRQ) Mood scales	Change negative automatic thoughts and beliefs about HF/NS, sleep and menopause Improve mood	Provide information about aetiology, causes and impacts of HF/NS and menopause Cognitive therapy Stress management
Behavioural reactions	Diaries or rating scales of behaviours	Improve relaxation skills Increase acceptance of HF/NS Increase self-efficacy in coping with HF/NS Change sleep habits	Paced breathing Behavioural experiments, e.g. communication and reducing avoidance CBT for sleep

WHY GROUP CBT?

Until recently hormone therapy (HT) has been the recommended medical treatment for hot flushes, and is an effective treatment for hot flushes (Archer et al. 2011). However, HT has been associated with a small but increased risk of breast cancer, thrombosis and stroke (Rossouw et al. 2002; Beral 2003). These findings have resulted in decreased HT use, with many women declining or discontinuing HT between 2002 and 2005 in the UK and the USA (Hersh et al. 2004; Menon et al. 2007; Sprague et al. 2012). The UK Committee on Safety of Medicines (2002) recommended that HT should be used for the treatment of menopausal symptoms only, and at low doses for limited time intervals, such as five years. Recent evidence suggests that HT is likely to be safer than was previously suggested (Schierbeck et al. 2012; de Villiers et al. 2013) and individual risk–benefit analysis is suggested with discussion between the woman and health provider, taking into account her preferences and individual circumstances (de Villiers et al. 2013). For example, women who have early menopause are advised to have HT up until the natural age of menopause, i.e. 50 years, and it is safe and beneficial for health to do so (Panay and Fenton 2008). A UK National Institute for Health and Care Excellence (NICE) guidance on 'Menopause: diagnosis and management of menopause' is due to report on the current available evidence of treatments in July 2015 (http://guidance.nice.org.uk/CG/Wave0/639).

As a result of the uncertainties about the safety of HT, there has been increased interest in the development of non-hormonal alternatives, and many women use over the counter treatments. Alternative medical treatments include selective serotonin and norepinephrine reuptake inhibitors (SSRI/SNRIs), clonidine and gabapentin. Studies of the effects of SSRIs suggest that they can reduce hot flushes, particularly for women who have had breast cancer, but their effects are variable in studies with non-cancer populations (Suvanto-Luukkonen et al. 2005; Carroll 2006). Recent systematic reviews of the evidence for the effectiveness of these treatments tend to conclude that SSRI/SNRIs, clonidine and gabapentin can reduce hot flushes but that side effects such as nausea, dry mouth and loss of libido, are commonly reported (Nelson et al. 2006; Rada et al. 2010). Similarly, there is little evidence to support the use of over the counter remedies, such as oil of evening primrose, vitamin E, wild yam and black cohosh (Nelson et al. 2006; Borrelli and Ernst 2010). Moreover, it is suggested that herbal medicinal products should be used with caution because some may interact with other medications (Pitkin 2012). Consequently, there is a need for effective and acceptable treatments to help women to manage menopausal symptoms (Kadakia et al. 2012).

Several small-scale studies (Stevenson and Delprato 1983; Freedman and Woodward 1992; Germaine and Freedman 1984; Irvin et al. 1996; Wijma et al. 1997) have shown that paced breathing (regular diaphragmatic breathing) and relaxation can result in decreases in hot flushes in samples of well women. Relaxation has also been shown to reduce the frequency and severity of hot flushes in the short term in a trial of 150 breast cancer patients (Fenlon et al. 2008).

We began to study the effectiveness of cognitive behaviour therapy (CBT) for menopausal hot flushes in a primary care setting (Hunter and Liao 1996) using a patient preference design to compare the effectiveness of CBT with HT (comparing no treatment (monitoring) versus HT versus CBT). A four-session (one to one, face to face) CBT intervention, combining psycho-education, relaxation and cognitive therapy, was offered to 24 women to help them cope with their flushes through learning to identify and modify triggers and exacerbators of hot flushes, using relaxation to reduce general levels of stress and using cognitive therapy to challenge overly negative thoughts and beliefs. Sessions focused on discussing the nature of hot flushes, as well as attitudes and beliefs about the menopause, with the aim of helping women to identify their automatic thoughts and reduce their distress by adopting strategies such as calming self-talk, challenging unhelpful beliefs, relaxation and breathing exercises. CBT and HT demonstrated comparable effectiveness, reducing the frequency of hot flushes by 50 per cent and those who had received CBT reported greater confidence in their ability to cope. There were no significant changes in the self-monitoring group. Compared with HT, CBT also appeared to enhance general mood by lowering levels of anxiety and depression. Subsequently, Keefer and Blanchard (2005) conducted a pilot study (n=19) of Group CBT (8 x 90 min sessions) and found significant reductions in the total number of hot flushes compared with a wait list control (delayed treatment group).

We then carried out a pilot study of Group CBT (6 x 90 min sessions) for 17 women with hot flushes following breast cancer treatments and found that the treatment was acceptable and led to significant reductions in hot flush frequency and problem-rating (extent to which they are problematic) (Hunter et al. 2009a). However, systematic reviews of psychosocial or mind–body interventions for menopausal symptoms (Tremblay et al. 2008; Innes et al. 2010) concluded that, while these interventions (including relaxation, yoga and cognitive behavioural interventions) are acceptable and there is some supportive evidence, further evaluation of treatment effects in high-quality randomised controlled trials are required.

MENOS 1 AND MENOS 2 TRIALS

Two randomised controlled trials of Group CBT have recently been completed for women who have hot flushes and night sweats following breast cancer treatment (MENOS 1 (Mann et al. 2012): comparing Group CBT versus usual care) and for healthy women (MENOS 2 (Ayers et al. 2011; Ayers et al. 2012): comparing Group CBT versus self-help CBT versus no treatment). These trials included both subjective and physiological measures (sternal skin conductance) of hot flushes and a measure of problem-rating or bothersomeness. Problem-rating is the most clinically relevant measure because it is associated with their impact on quality of life and help-seeking (Ayers and Hunter 2012) and is measured using the Hot Flush Rating Scale (HFRS) (Hunter and Liao 1995; see Figure 1.3, page 14). Results of both trials show that these CBT interventions are effective in reducing the impact, or problem-rating, of hot flushes and have additional benefits to mood and quality of life. In MENOS 2 the group and self-help interventions were equally effective in reducing how problematic hot flushes were rated, but Group CBT had more additional benefits to mood and quality of life.

MENOS 1 compared Group CBT with usual care for women with problematic hot flushes following breast cancer treatments. Ninety six women who were experiencing problematic hot flushes (minimum ten problematic flushes a week) following breast cancer treatment were randomised to receive either usual care (n=49) or Group CBT plus usual care (n=47). Assessments were conducted at baseline, 9 and 26 weeks post-randomisation. Group CBT significantly reduced hot flush problem-rating at 9 weeks post-randomisation compared with usual care, and improvements were maintained at 26 weeks. At 26 weeks, 78 per cent of women in the CBT arm had a clinically significant reduction in hot flush problem-rating (change score greater than 2 points from baseline) compared with 33 per cent (95 per cent CI: 20–48 per cent) in the usual care arm. Both CBT and usual care groups reduced frequency of hot flushes; those having Group CBT reported fewer night sweats at 26 weeks than usual care but the difference was not significant. In this study women having usual care were quite well supported, having access to cancer support services. There were significant improvements in mood, sleep, and quality of life for Group CBT participants compared with usual care.

In MENOS 2, 140 women having problematic hot flushes were randomised to Group CBT, self-help CBT or no treatment control (NTC). Group CBT and self-help CBT both had significantly reduced hot flush problem-rating at 6 weeks and at 26 weeks. In total, 65 per cent of Group CBT and 73 per cent of self-help participants reported clinically significant improvements of two points or more on the hot flush problem-rating scale following treatment and these changes were maintained at the follow-up assessment at 26 weeks post-randomisation. In addition, both Group and self-help CBT led to significantly fewer night sweats (frequency) at 26 weeks. Significant improvements in mood and quality of life were evident at 6 weeks and improved emotional and physical functioning for Group CBT at 26 weeks.

We also found that there were small but significant improvements in memory and concentration for those women who had CBT compared with those who had not, and this was the case in both trials, i.e. for well women going through the menopause transition (Ayers et al. 2012) and for women who had hot flushes following treatment for breast cancer (Mann et al. 2012). In general the evidence suggests that stress and mood, as well as hot flushes and night sweats, are associated with subjective reports of memory problems (Henderson 2009; Mitchell and Woods 2011), so the improvement in flushes and mood might have also influenced experience of concentration and memory.

For both MENOS 1 and 2 trials, CBT resulted in positive changes in hot flush beliefs and behaviours, and hot flush beliefs have subsequently been found to be the main mediators of improvement following CBT (Chilcot et al. 2014; Norton et al. 2014). When we examined the physiological measure of hot flushes (sternal skin conductance) we found that there were significant reductions in physiologically measured hot flushes for women who had received CBT compared with the control group (Stefanopoulou and Hunter 2013). Interestingly, this was the case for well women in MENOS 2 but not for women who had had breast cancer (MENOS 1). A possible explanation for this finding is that the majority of women in the MENOS 1 trial were having Tamoxifen or other endocrine medication, which can exacerbate hot flushes. Nevertheless, CBT was effective for breast cancer survivors who were premenopausal at diagnosis, for those who had had chemotherapy, and for those who were having endocrine treatment, such as Tamoxifen (Chilcot et al. 2014).

The effectiveness of CBT for younger women, who were premenopausal when they developed breast cancer, was supported by a Dutch study comparing Group CBT with exercise, exercise plus CBT and usual care (Duijts et al. 2012). Using the same Group CBT format as MENOS 1, we found that women who received CBT reported significant improvements in hot flush problem-rating compared with usual care, while those who received exercise alone did not.

We carried out qualitative interviews with random samples of approximately 20 per cent of participants at the end of MENOS 1 and 2 trials to find out how women viewed the treatment. The results of MENOS 1 qualitative analysis (Balabanovic et al. 2012) suggest that the women gained confidence and ability to cope with hot flushes and night sweats; they described gaining control over the physical symptoms using paced breathing and cognitive and behavioural strategies and they found the group context helpful in terms of normalising their problems and in motivating them in homework tasks as well as providing support. The accounts from women in the MENOS 2 trial were similar (Balabanovic et al. 2013). Key factors mentioned were a restored sense of control (experienced on a number of different levels and often facilitated by paced breathing) and acceptance. Many women noticed that they attended differently to their hot flushes, i.e. they may have been having hot flushes but did not notice them. Perhaps reflecting the skills learning involved, the beneficial effects of the treatment in some cases extended beyond management of menopausal symptoms. In general Group CBT had greater popular appeal relative to self-help CBT; women valued the experiential aspects of the group including meeting others in a similar situation, experiencing support and normalisation.

ASSESSMENT FOR GROUP CBT

Assessment includes a psychosocial and health assessment, as well as assessment of hot flushes and preparation for Group CBT. When selecting group members it is important to remember that the programme requires a reasonable level of understanding of spoken and written English so this will need to be clarified. Materials are currently only available in English but are likely to be translated in the future. Women who are primarily seeking psychological support or treatment for other problems, such as depression, anxiety or bereavement, should be encouraged to seek other services, since although mood generally improves following Group CBT for hot flushes this is not the prime target, and primary care services are available that will provide more appropriate interventions. It is helpful to take details of the woman's doctor (General Practitioner, GP) and/or other health care professionals and to ask the woman's permission to inform the GP that she is attending the programme.

We suggest the following inclusion and exclusion criteria are screened for during the assessment:

- Having problematic hot flushes: in our research women had on average 60 hot flushes a week and problem-ratings of 6/10 on average, which typically reduced to an average of 3/10 after treatment.
- Hot flushes or night sweats are the main problem for which they are seeking help.
- Adequate use of spoken and written English.
- Not suffering from major psychiatric or physical health problems that would make participation in the groups difficult.
- Ability to travel and make time commitments.
- Willing to participate in groups.

Assessments typically last for 40 to 60 minutes and can be carried out face to face or by telephone. We usually include the following:

- Socio-demographic information.
- A brief medical and psychiatric history, including past and current medication for menopausal symptoms; for women who have had breast cancer, information about cancer stage and treatment would be elicited.
- Clinical interview covering history of menopausal symptoms, treatment and duration and experience of symptoms, and psychosocial assessment including mood, current concerns and lifestyle.
- Questionnaire measures of hot flushes, mood and health related quality of life. Several questionnaires are suggested below but these can be tailored to the needs of the particular setting:
    - The Hot Flush Rating Scale (Hunter and Liao 1995) is a short scale which measures hot flush and night sweat Frequency and Problem-rating (the average of three items including distress, extent to which they are problematic and interfere with daily routine). It is Problem-rating that is the main outcome measure

Hot flush frequency:

1. How often have you had hot flushes in the past week?

Please estimate: ________ times each day, or ________ times each week

2. If you have night sweats, how often have they woken you up in the past week?

Please estimate: ________ times each night, or ________ times each week

Hot Flush Problem-Rating:

Please circle a notch on each scale to indicate how your flushes/sweats have been during the past week:

3. To what extent do you regard your flushes/sweats as a problem?

No problem at all 1 2 3 4 5 6 7 8 9 10 Very much a problem

4. How distressed do you feel about your hot flushes?

Not distressed at all 1 2 3 4 5 6 7 8 9 10 Very distressed indeed

5. How much do your hot flushes interfere with your daily routine?

Not at all 1 2 3 4 5 6 7 8 9 10 Very much indeed

Add up the numbers of hot flushes and night sweats in the past week which gives your

Hot flush frequency total score = ...

and add up the scores on numbers 3, 4 and 5 and divide by 3. This will give you your

Problem-Rating score = ... which is the main measure that we aim to change.

Figure 1.3 Hot Flush Rating Scale: frequency and problem-rating (Hunter and Liao 1995)

that we aim to change. This scale can be given out at assessment and at the end of the treatment. The scale is shown in Figure 1.3 and can be downloaded at: www.routledge.com/9781138026155.

- Daily diary recording of hot flushes is helpful to monitor change during the treatment. Daily diaries are regarded as more reliable because the flushes can be recorded at the time. However, night sweats are typically estimated the next morning. These can include frequency or frequency plus a rating of severity and are usually given out at assessment and weekly during the group sessions (Figure 1.4).
- The Hot Flush Beliefs Scale (Rendall et al. 2008) is a 27-item scale developed using factor analysis and has three subscales: (i) beliefs about HF in social context (e.g. everyone is looking at me), (ii) beliefs about coping/control of hot flushes (e.g. when I have a HF I think they will never end), and (iii) beliefs about night sweats and sleep (e.g. if I have NS I'll never get back to sleep).

Week 1 2 3 4 5 6 7 Date:

	Monday	***Tuesday***	***Wednesday***	***Thursday***	***Friday***	***Saturday***	***Sunday***
1–6am							
6–9am							
9–12pm							
12–2pm							
2–4pm							
4–6pm							
6–8pm							
8–10pm							
10–12am							

Hot Flushes: Place a √ in the box
Relaxation: Place an X in the box
Night Sweats: Place an o in the box

Figure 1.4 Hot flush daily diary

- The Hot Flush Behaviour Scale (Hunter et al. 2011) was developed using factor analysis and includes three subscales measuring, (i) positive coping behaviour, e.g. accepting HF/NS, using breathing and calming responses; (ii) avoidance behaviour, and (iii) cooling behaviours, such as fanning oneself.
- The Menopause Representation Questionnaire (MRQ) (Hunter and O'Dea 2001) provides a measure of attribution of symptoms to the menopause, as well as positive and negative beliefs about the menopause.
- Questionnaires developed for mid aged women include the Women's Health Questionnaire (Hunter 1992), which measures mood, somatic symptoms, sleep, sexual functioning, and the Greene Climacteric Scale (Greene 1998), which has subscales assessing somatic, psychological, vasomotor, and sexual functioning. However other standardised measures of anxiety, depressed mood, stress and/or quality of life can be used depending on the setting.

- Provide the rationale for the treatment, for example: 'There is some evidence that hot flushes can be made worse by stress and can be precipitated by specific factors such as certain foods and drinks, and we know that paced breathing and relaxation can help reduce the impact of them. There is also some evidence that women can learn ways of coping with hot flushes (using cognitive and behavioural strategies) so that the symptoms become less troublesome. We are offering a combination of these treatments in groups so that women can also gain support from one another.'

- Description of group intervention (6 x 1.5 hour sessions or the format can be modified to change the number of sessions to 4 x 2 hour sessions) and expectations of treatment, including ground rules, importance of homework, completion of measures and diaries and attendance at sessions. Follow-up sessions or telephone follow-up appointments can be arranged three and or six months after treatment.

Assessment interviews are helpful in order to prepare women for Group CBT. Provision of information about the time commitments, dates of the group sessions, content of the groups and homework tasks is important so that women can make a commitment to attend the programme or not. Some ground rules of the Group CBT can be discussed at assessment session, although they are also repeated in the first session:

- Confidentiality.
- Focus on being constructive.
- Sharing group time and taking turns.
- Not obliged to do anything you don't want to but encouraged to try.
- Agree to commit to attend all sessions but if unforeseen events, e.g. if unwell, then call beforehand.
- Some issues not the focus of the group.

Some people prefer not to meet in groups so we have developed a self-help form of the treatment that is effective (MENOS 2) and is available as an alternative in book form and as an e-book (Hunter and Smith 2013). We have tended to offer separate groups for women who have undergone breast cancer treatments versus well women who have gone through a natural menopause, because group members are likely to be able to support each other more easily when they have a shared experience. But this is not essential. Similarly, the programme includes separate sections that may have more or less relevance to different groups of women. If for practical reasons these groups (women who have and those who have not had cancer) need to be included together, then steps can be taken to cover the relevant themes in the groups.

Other differences between women include age at menopause and type of menopause (induced by surgery or medication or 'natural'). For younger group members (well women or breast cancer patients), in their early 40s or younger, who perhaps will not have anticipated that menopause would be an issue for them at this point in their lives, careful preparation is needed. Ideally, a separate early menopause group, or younger breast cancer survivors groups could be conducted to meet the needs of this group of women. However, limited resources often mean that this is not possible. Therefore, the facilitator can discuss this issue with the participant prior to the group, as well as monitoring the situation during the sessions. Women who have surgical or chemically induced menopause often experience more hot flushes following a rapid withdrawal of oestrogen. They may benefit from discussing the reasons for their menopause in the group. In our experience a mixed group of women can work well if they have been prepared, since each member is likely to discover other similarities between themselves and other group members.

SETTING UP GROUP CBT SESSIONS

Before assessing women for Group CBT you will need to plan the following:

- Place – a room large enough for 10–12 people to sit in a semicircle in a venue that is easily accessible by public transport.
- Time – a regular time each week with time for preparation included. We found late afternoon or early evening to be a good time.
- Group leaders – ideally, having two people, a trained group leader and a trainee or volunteer, works well and is a useful training experience.
- Number of participants – between 6 and 10 is optimal.
- Inclusion/exclusion criteria see page 13.
- Materials: CDs, handouts, projector for PowerPoint slides, questionnaires, drinks (water is usually sufficient).

Some training in group work and regular supervision for group leaders is essential. We have identified some common issues that can arise when running groups; these can be discussed prior to the programme and in the training and supervision:

- People not listening, distracting others.
- People not saying anything.
- People being disruptive, very emotional, aggressive.
- Group member trying to be the leader.
- None attendance or late arrivals.
- People not doing homework.
- Not covering the material and running out of time.

Most of these can be prevented by careful preparation by group leaders and taking time to discuss the group process following each group (group facilitator/leader and volunteer) and during supervision.

Some helpful strategies to consider include:

- Deal with practical issues and prepare for the group.
- Rehearse the timing and roles.
- Prepare participants at assessment interview.
- Have clear ground rules.
- Present clear rationale and agree goals at assessment/session one.
- Keep to time.

Women are often understandably quite anxious when joining a group and can express this in a variety of ways, for example, withdrawing and avoiding participation, or sometimes trying to control the group by talking a lot and taking a leading role. Careful timing is very important because there is a lot of material to cover and unexpected issues might arise which might take a bit more time, so for this reason times are allocated to each task or section of each group. Allocating roles to the main group facilitator (running the Group CBT etc.) and student/volunteer (preparing room, collecting questionnaires, helping when women are discussing goals in pairs, giving out homework sheets, writing on flip charts and keeping a strict eye on the timing of the sessions) helps to break up the sessions and helps them to run efficiently.

Some things to consider in terms of roles and responsibilities so that the sessions run smoothly:

- Prepare for each session with co-leader.
- Be enthusiastic and use the group to motivate.
- Practise giving relaxation/paced breathing instructions and make time for this in each session.
- Review homework and collect questionnaires at the beginning of each session.
- At the end of each session explain homework and give out handouts.
- Give out and collect questionnaires at the end of sessions.
- Debrief with co-leader and make notes after the session and set aside time to prepare for the next session.

During the group sessions we make use of several different exercises that help to encourage individuals and set the scene for participation in the group discussions:

- Go round: introductions, problem description.
- Presentations (PowerPoint slides) and discussion: cognitions and CBT model.
- Brainstorm (flip chart, note taker): precipitants, cognitions and behaviours, menopause beliefs.
- Pairs/subgroup discussion groups with group feedback: stress-reducing goals, sleep goals.
- Direct experience: relaxation, paced breathing.
- Role-play: having a hot flush and using paced breathing and cognitions.

In the following chapters each session is described in detail. Each session begins with a session summarising timings for the different sections. The sessions are in the 6 x 1.5 hourly format, but it is possible to run groups in 4 sessions of 2 hours by combining some sessions: 1, 2+3, 4+5, 6. We include information and discussion of the aspects of the intervention with examples of explanations that can be used during the groups. Reading through the chapters before group sessions will provide background information so that the group sessions can be delivered focusing on the specific group activities that are outlined in the summary. In our experience the sessions become easier to deliver with practice, so that once the programme has been running for two or more intakes the group facilitator gains confidence and skills. We have found the groups enjoyable and rewarding to run too. As mentioned earlier, fixing supervision time is important to manage discussions in the groups and any questions that arise.

Handouts and copies of the PowerPoint slides are included in Chapter 8. The Hot Flush Rating Scale, Weekly Diaries, PowerPoint slides and relaxation/breathing exercises can be downloaded from:

www.routledge.com/9781138026155.

For information about training sessions please email: Myra.hunter@kcl.ac.uk

2

Session 1: Psycho-education and the cognitive behavioural model

SUMMARY OF SESSION 1

- Introduction – ground rules for group participants, aims of the group including summary of rationale for Group cognitive behaviour therapy (CBT), and a brief outline of group sessions. (Handout 1) (5 mins)
- Group introductions – each woman introduces herself by talking briefly about her menopausal symptoms, what is most difficult for her, and what her goals are for the group. (20 mins)
- Psycho-education about the physiological mechanisms of hot flushes and night sweats and cognitive behavioural model. (Handout 2) (20 mins total) To include:
    - The thermo-neutral zone (give copy of diagram) (5 mins)
    - Emotions, thoughts and behaviours that accompany hot flushes and night sweats (group task where facilitator completes CBT model on flip chart) (10–15 mins)
    - A summary of the cognitive behavioural model of menopausal symptoms, and treatment rationale. (Handout 3)
- Discussion of precipitants – brainstorm on flip chart. (10 mins)
  Provide information about common precipitants, e.g. coffee, tea, rushing, hot rooms and write down on flip chart.
- Relaxation introduction with focus on paced breathing. (30 mins)
  Discuss experience of relaxation. Provide relaxation CD or URL for homework. Suggest daily practice in quiet room at specified time. Group discussion of potential barriers to practise and how to overcome them. Encourage group support to practise.
- Homework with debrief discussion of any questions. (5 mins)
  Homework: to be aware of precipitants and to make a note on the daily diary and daily practice of relaxation and breathing, which can be noted on the daily diary.

Photocopying this summary and having a copy for the facilitator and assistant can help timekeeping when running the session.

SESSION 1

In our experience, the first session tends to be the most important session for ensuring that participants return week after week. Our studies demonstrated that if people returned for the second session they were highly likely to attend sessions through to the end of the intervention. Highlighting that the intervention is evidence-based and involves the implementation of a combination of effective strategies is paramount, as participants have often tried other medical and non-medical approaches that have not worked too well, or have had side effects. It is helpful for the facilitator to describe the intervention as a self-management strategy that reduces the impact that flushes may have on the lives of the women rather than a 'cure'. S/he will need to reinforce the idea that the intervention is not designed to eliminate flushes completely so that initial expectations are realistic. Ideally this will have been discussed prior to group attendance, i.e. during an assessment interview. However, the facilitator may wish to outline the potential benefits that have been reported by people who have completed the intervention; for example, an increase in coping, reduction in the impact that hot flushes have on quality of life and improved sleep. The aim is to encourage group members to adopt a realistic but optimistic approach at a time when they are likely to be sceptical or disheartened by numerous previous attempts to manage hot flushes.

INITIAL GROUP INTERACTIONS AND WHAT TO EXPECT

Participants may be somewhat apprehensive initially at the prospect of attending a group intervention. Common concerns include meeting new people and talking openly with strangers or in front of a group or saying something wrong or looking foolish. The facilitator can acknowledge and normalise this anxiety from the outset by reassuring participants that there are no incorrect answers and that everyone's contribution is highly valued. Setting ground rules can also help to reduce anxiety and establish a receptive and collaborative atmosphere. Uncertainties about how a psychological approach might help a physical symptom may also lead to scepticism; the facilitator can acknowledge that this is a common concern but that the approach will be described in this session.

At the end of this session, the facilitator can check if attendees have any anxieties now about the group and provide reassurance or positive feedback; this can make the difference between the person continuing to participate in the intervention or not returning due to feeling embarrassed. This is particularly relevant if someone has become emotional during the session. Our experience of first sessions is that group members occasionally become emotional when introducing themselves and discussing experiences relating to menopause and midlife and negative perceptions of self. For breast cancer patients, the psychological impact of the cancer diagnosis, as well as the demanding treatment regime that resulted in distressing menopausal symptoms, can result in feelings of anger or hopelessness. While other participants are likely to communicate support, which can help the group to form preliminary relationships, the facilitator should take the opportunity to reassure participants that emotional reactions are common and understandable, particularly as participants may have not previously verbalised these concerns to others. The group should be encouraged to keep personal information within the boundaries of the group. The facilitator can encourage this by highlighting the confidentiality agreement discussed as part of the ground rules.

Session 1, Slide 1

What will you need?

Flip chart and pens
Homework sheets 1–3
A folder for each client containing hot flush weekly diary and hot flush rating scale
Relaxation CD (these can be downloaded on to CDs for participants or they can use the website address themselves)
A watch or clock

Agenda

For each session, it is helpful to have an agenda prepared and written on the flip chart for participants to see. This is good practice in any cognitive behavioural work to set the scene for the session and it enables everyone involved to ensure that everything is covered. Additionally, it provides boundaries during group discussions to keep discussions within the topic and within an approximate time frame.

Session 1 example agenda

Introductions and ground rules
Your experience of menopausal symptoms and goals
The physiology of hot flushes
The role of thoughts, feelings and behaviour
Identifying what brings them on and makes them worse
Relaxation and paced breathing

Introduction to Group CBT for hot flushes, including ground rules for group participants, aims of the group, and a brief outline of group sessions and summarise rationale. (Handout 1) (5 mins)

The facilitator introduces themselves and their professional background and asks the group members to introduce themselves by name. Having name stickers can be useful.

Session 1, Slides 2 and 3

General practical information, such as the group dates and times, the location of the toilets and what refreshments (if any) will be available to the group can also be explained. Establishing the boundaries of the group is essential to help people to feel safe to share information. The ground rules can be prepared and presented to the group for additions and comments. For example:

- Confidentiality
- Focus on being constructive
- Sharing group time and taking turns – listening
- Not obliged to do anything you don't want to but encouraged to try
- Agree to commit to attend all sessions but if unforeseen events, e.g. if unwell, then call beforehand
- Some issues not the focus of the group.

Then spend a few minutes introducing the aims of the group sessions, including the emphasis on self-management skills, by running through Slide 3 and using the following text. Give out Handout 1 – Outline of group sessions.

Sample introduction to treatment

This is a six session programme based on a combination of non-medical treatments that have been found, in previous research, to help women to manage menopausal symptoms. These are based on a well-developed therapy called cognitive behavioural therapy (CBT). The cognitive part looks at the way we think about the symptoms and how this affects the way we feel. The behavioural part looks at ways we can change our behaviour to promote wellbeing and coping with hot flushes.

Getting the most out of the groups will be down to you. We will be asking you to do homework between sessions so that you have the chance to practise what we have been covering in the sessions. Sometimes it is difficult to find time to spend on ourselves so do think about how you can manage to find time each week to put some of the things we will be covering in the group into practice. Undertaking the relaxation and other tasks in the programme will help you to feel more in control of what is happening to you and is likely to have a positive effect on other parts of your life as well. Be patient if you find it hard initially and try not to get discouraged. If you miss one or two days, it doesn't mean you have to start again. Simply decide that today will be different and you will find the time again. Committing yourself and finding the time to work on your own needs is worthwhile and ultimately rewarding. We encourage you to offer this time to yourself and to persevere even when it seems difficult. Our work in the past suggests that small changes can make a big difference.

Breast Cancer Patient Specific

The period following breast cancer can be challenging as you come to terms with your experience of illness. You may be trying to resume normal activities while experiencing ongoing physical symptoms such as menopausal symptoms. This can also be a time of uncertainty with worries about dealing with the present and the future. This programme is designed to help you to manage these physical symptoms experienced following breast cancer treatments, as well as to provide information to promote wellbeing and health, in particular looking after yourself and reducing stress. Later in the sessions you will have the opportunity to discuss with other group members any issues you feel haven't been discussed in the groups but which may be important to you following breast cancer treatment.

Menopause experiences and goals – each woman talks briefly about her menopausal symptoms, what is most difficult for her and what her goals are for the group. (20 mins)

Session 1, Slide 4

Following the introduction, group members are invited to briefly tell the group about their experience of menopause and what brings them to the group; this can be done by going round each person in turn. By the end of the exercise, each person will be aware of the following information about group members:

- What is your experience of menopause?
- What would you like to change/what are your goals for the group?

It is helpful to record goals on a flip chart to refer back to in the final session. That way, anything that has not been addressed can be discussed during the 'free-discussion' in the last session (Session 6). Some examples of goals from our groups are:

- To control the hot flushes and night sweats
- To improve my sleeping patterns

- To know what triggers my hot flushes
- Understand the emotional aspects of menopausal symptoms
- Coping skills for dealing with hot flushes
- Relaxation
- To try and reduce hot flushes.

PSYCHO-EDUCATION

Provide information about menopause and the physiology of hot flushes (Handout 2) and the cognitive behavioural model of menopausal symptoms, which shows the relationships between physical changes and thoughts, mood, behaviour and lifestyle (Handout 3).

Session 1, Slides 5 and 6

Menopause

The facilitator provides a brief synopsis of menopause and invites questions (Slide 5), adapting it according to whether the group are well women experiencing natural menopause, or women experiencing symptoms following treatment for breast cancer. For menopausal well-women, there is likely to be an emphasis on the psychosocial, age or life transitions they are going through as well as the physical changes. Typically this can raise questions about attitudes and beliefs about menopause, ageing, identity and roles, as well as plans for the future. This life transition can result in uncertainty but also possible benefits as they move onto a new life stage.

For participants with breast cancer, the focus will be initially on acknowledging their experience of breast cancer diagnosis and treatment as well as the potential uncertainty and subsequent anxieties they may currently be experiencing.

The physiology of hot flushes

Providing information about the physiology of hot flushes and the thermo-neutral zone is a vital part of understanding and managing symptoms. Having a 'scientific explanation', which highlights the role of stress in relation to hot flushes can encourage participants to engage in stress management, as well as promoting calm cognitive and behavioural responses. It also normalises their experiences. A sample explanation is outlined on this page. Women are usually very interested in the thermo-neutral zone diagram and explanation and understanding of why they are experiencing flushes, so ensure adequate time is allowed for discussion.

Explaining the physiology of hot flushes to the group

Everybody has a thermo-neutral zone (hot flush threshold), which is the range of temperatures that your body can experience without having to actively regulate. Body temperature can go up or down and your body adapts to this without having to sweat to cool you down, or shiver to warm you up. A woman with no menopausal symptoms would be shown in the top part of the diagram.

Because hormones and body temperature control are linked, the hot flush threshold becomes narrower following the menopause, and following types of breast cancer treatment, due to changes in oestrogen levels. Therefore there is a smaller range of temperature change that your body can experience before regulation (sweating and/or shivering) starts. The same changes that your body could tolerate before may now trigger hot flushes and night sweats. This is shown in the second part of the diagram.

Stress also affects the hot flush threshold so that with ongoing stress the zone narrows. Previous research suggests that being stressed or anxious tends to raise the frequency and intensity of hot flushes overall. The body will naturally adjust to the hormonal changes over time and eventually the hot flushes/night sweats stop. This is a gradual process.

The cognitive behavioural model

Session 1, Slide 7

Cognitive and behavioural factors are presented first (Slide 7) and then these are discussed within cognitive behavioural model of menopausal symptoms (Slide 8).

Using a flip chart with a CBT model prepared (shown in Slide 7), the facilitator can introduce participants to the model by recording thoughts, feelings and behaviours associated with hot flushes or night sweats in the relevant part of the diagram. The aim is to identify physiological reactions, thoughts, feelings and behaviours during hot flushes. Initially it is helpful for the facilitator to focus on one component at a time rather than attempting to link up cycles of thoughts, feelings and behaviour, as the aim here is to introduce cognitive behavioural components as a new concept rather than start making links. Once the diagram is completed, the facilitator may ask participants if they notice anything about the diagram, particularly the emotions, thoughts and behaviours.

The facilitator may also give the group an example to work through (see below) if they have any initial difficulties with this task, although it is preferable to use examples from the group, which may be referred back to at later sessions.

Example of a woman who may be busy trying to get back into her work but is *experiencing hot flushes* and *thinks that others are looking at her critically* when she has hot flushes. For example, she may *feel worried and low* and therefore *avoid meeting up with people* which then makes her *feel worse* about herself and *more stressed*.

There are occasionally participants who already respond calmly to hot flushes both cognitively and behaviourally. For example, one participant identified the *thoughts* '*This will pass soon*' and '*This is natural and other women go through it*'. Consequently she did not report any strong emotional reactions. She would then *behave* calmly by remaining in the situation and took simple steps to cool off such as removing layers and using a fan. This can be used as a helpful example that demonstrates the cognitive behavioural model equally as well as more negative responses. The facilitator can add it to the flip chart in a different pen colour next to the other examples to illustrate how calmer *cognitive* responses resulted in calmer *feelings* and *behaviour*.

Session 1, Slide 8

The CBT model includes the relationships between the physical experience of a hot flush and concurrent thoughts, mood, behaviour and lifestyle. This enables the facilitator to acknowledge the important role of physiological factors and avoid potential misunderstandings that a psychological intervention may imply that participants' experiences are 'all in the mind'. Presenting the diagram of the cognitive behavioural model of menopausal symptoms provides a rationale for the Group CBT, which the facilitator can then link in with specific interventions covered in this manual.

Session 1, Slide 9

The main elements of the treatment are then described and shown on Slide 9.

Treatment rationale

Previous research suggests that by making changes and modifications to thinking and behaviour, women can develop strategies that help them to feel more in control of hot flushes when they occur and can reduce the impact that hot flushes have on their life if they are able to implement and maintain changes.

So while the reduction in oestrogen leads to the narrowing of the hot flush threshold, managing stress and making changes to your lifestyle, including modifying triggers, can help to modify the impact of this. Practising relaxation is also a powerful way to reduce feelings of stress and manage hot flushes when practised regularly. In particular, research into a type of breathing called paced breathing has demonstrated that this promotes feelings of calmness if practised regularly and when implemented at the onset of a hot flush. Stress can also be addressed using a range of psychological and behavioural strategies that we will be finding out more about in Session 2. Because thinking and behavioural responses to hot flushes or night sweats can influence whether women feel they can cope with them or not, making changes to thinking and behavioural responses can lead to improved coping strategies and feelings of control. Therefore, working on changing thinking and behavioural responses can reduce the impact of troublesome hot flushes. Cognitive behaviour therapy helps people to spot overly negative or catastrophic responses to hot flushes and night sweats. By recognising particular patterns of thinking, we can instead use more adaptive or neutral patterns of thinking which we will learn about initially in the stress session and apply specifically to hot flushes in Session 3.

We can also apply this cognitive behavioural work to night sweats. Because night sweats also impact on sleep and lead to daytime tiredness, we will also be doing some work on sleep and looking at minor changes you may be able to make to improve your sleep quality and reduce worry about being woken by night sweats.

DISCUSSION OF PRECIPITANTS AND BRAINSTORM ON FLIP CHART

Discuss common *precipitants*, e.g. coffee, tea, rushing, hot rooms and write them down on the flip chart. The aim is to encourage participants to identify and monitor triggers as homework and then in future sessions, if lifestyle related triggers are identified, they can make changes to aspects of their daily routine accordingly. This introduces an element of control to managing hot flushes. The facilitator can introduce this section by citing previous research into triggers and highlighting the variation in individual experiences of triggers. For homework, group members should be aware of precipitants and make a note in their daily diary.

Session 1, Slide 10

Group members can discuss in pairs (or in the group) any specific triggers to hot flushes or night sweats they are already aware of. The facilitator can note these on a flip chart. While women may already be aware of some triggers, the homework task introduces the idea of monitoring as an important CBT skill. Once they have made suggestions, the facilitator can present Slide 10, showing common triggers that are likely to confirm or complement the experiences of the group.

Introducing the role of triggers

Studies of women with menopausal symptoms suggest that about 50 per cent of hot flushes may be triggered by a particular event or activity. We have found that women vary a lot in what triggers their hot flushes and some women can't identify any triggers. So this week it would be helpful if you could note down anything that happens just before the flush begins to help in understanding your hot flushes, which is the first step in managing them.

RELAXATION INTRODUCTION AND GROUP RELAXATION EXERCISE

Gentle tensing and relaxing of muscles through the body and focus on paced breathing.

Session 1, Slide 11

There is evidence that relaxation and paced breathing can reduce the impact of hot flushes in well women and women who are recovering from breast cancer. Participants develop relaxation skills in several stages over the course of the intervention, beginning with general relaxation and moving towards implementing these during hot flushes. Initially, the focus is on introducing relaxation by helping group members to be aware of breathing and introduce progressive muscle relaxation. As they become skilled at relaxing, the focus shifts to breathing during a hot flush and switching their attentional focus to their breathing. Before starting the guided relaxation task, the facilitator should emphasise the following points:

- Relaxation and paced breathing have been found to reduce the impact of hot flushes and night sweats.
- Relaxation and paced breathing is a **skill** that requires **practice**.
- Initially participants might find relaxation quite difficult. This is normal and will become easier the more they practise.

The aim is to practise every day if possible. Participants are likely to need encouragement to make time to do relaxation, particularly if they lead busy or stressful lives. Mentioning the thermo-neutral zone and the impact of stress on this can motivate even the busiest of people to incorporate relaxation into their routine. The first session is a full 15 minute relaxation using body scan, tension and relaxation of areas of the body and focus of attention on breathing. A CD (or downloadable recording) is provided which contains the relaxation and breathing exercise. The facilitator should encourage participants to practise to develop relaxation skills.

Relaxation instructions (to be rehearsed and read out)

Relaxation involves learning a skill – you get better at it with practice so it helps to do the exercise every day at a regular time for 15 minutes. When you feel a flush coming on you can apply the relaxation response by relaxing your shoulders and arms, focusing on your breathing and letting the flush flow over you . . .

I am going to talk you through a 15 minute relaxation exercise. You can listen to this in a comfortable chair, or lying down. Make sure that you are in a quiet room free from interruptions (turn off phones etc.) and loosen any tight clothing. First just notice your body (body scan) – notice your body resting on the chair, notice your body from your head gradually down to your toes. If your mind drifts to thoughts or wanders don't worry just let the thought float through your mind and gently pass by – (imagery e.g. just like a cloud moving across the sky), and return to your body and your breathing.

Breathing: Relaxed breathing is gentle breathing from your stomach . . . your ribcage hardly needs to move . . . just feel the breath being drawn into your stomach . . . passing across the back of your throat. Push your stomach out slightly with each breath and as you breathe out feel yourself relaxing in to the chair. Just focus your attention on your breathing as you relax . . . with each breath feeling calm and relaxed.

Next we are going to relax main muscle groups in the body by first tensing them for a few seconds and then letting go and relaxing. By feeling the difference between tension and relaxation you can learn to detect tension and relax more easily.

Hands and arms . . . tense and relax . . . feel relaxation flowing down your arms to your hands. Breathing . . .

Shoulders, face and neck . . . tense and relax . . . relaxation flowing down from shoulders to arms and hands . . . arms feel heavy on the chair . . . an effort to move . . . Breathing . . .

Stomach . . . tense and relax . . . breathing . . . as breathe out stomach feels more relaxed.

Buttocks, legs and feet . . . tense and relax . . . breathe . . .

Now that we have worked through all the main parts of the body, I'd like you to focus on your breathing again and just let your body relax just a little more with each breath . . . feel yourself resting in the chair . . . it would be an effort to move . . . while you are relaxing you might want to think about a place that you have been which is pleasant for you . . . by a river or lying in the sun or maybe just watching something peaceful . . . notice the sounds, colours and the feeling of being in this calm place and spend a few minutes letting your thoughts and your body feel calm and peaceful.

(Few minutes)

Now slowly begin to be aware of where you are. When you are ready stretch your toes, feet and legs . . . then your arms and hands . . . and slowly open your eyes. Try to keep the relaxed feeling with you as you continue with your day, and notice your body and your breathing from time to time as you go about your activities.

When you have a hot flush take a breath, relax your shoulders arms and hands and let the flush and the relaxation flow through your body . . . notice your breathing and relax your body with each out breath.

For relaxation during the session, the facilitator can dim the lights, and try to make comfortable seating available. While hospital environments may not be ideal, this can be turned to an advantage in that the participants will eventually be aiming to implement relaxation and specifically paced breathing in stressful environments and uncomfortable surroundings during a hot flush.

HOMEWORK AND DEBRIEF DISCUSSION OF ANY QUESTIONS

At the end of the relaxation, group members are asked to feed back their reactions to the relaxation briefly. Within the first session, the most common feedback is that participants found it difficult to keep their attention focused on their breathing. Those who already do relaxation or practise meditation can reinforce the facilitator's message that they used to find this difficult but it became easier with practice. The facilitator can prompt this by checking around with people at the beginning.

Session 1, Slide 12

Homework

Group members are asked to do the following homework:

- Note down hot flushes and night sweats and any identified precipitants/triggers in the daily diary.
- Practise relaxation for 15–20 minutes on a daily basis if possible and note in diary.

The final few minutes can be set aside to check participants have understood the homework, to answer any questions and to give out handouts and diaries.

3

Session 2: Stress management, improving wellbeing and identifying precipitants

SUMMARY OF SESSION 2

- Review homework – look at diaries and discuss precipitants of hot flushes. Encourage group members to consider specific lifestyle changes to modify precipitants. (20 mins)
- Stress management and improving wellbeing – the focus of this session is to help women to reduce stress, improve wellbeing and also to deal with fatigue. (Handouts 4–6) (45 mins)

  Present information about the importance of reducing stress using a CBT approach as part of hot flush management: managing anxious thinking arising from stress, engaging in regular exercise (e.g. walking), pacing activities, engaging in pleasant activities (Handout 4), problem-solving (Handout 5) and set specific concrete individual goals for each person in pairs (Handout 6), and then feedback goals to the group.
- Discuss relaxation homework and encourage practice by discussion of barriers and how to overcome them. Group relaxation exercise. Tensing and relaxing muscles through the body and focus on paced breathing. (15 mins)
- Homework: To implement stress management goals, e.g. introduce a change in behaviour towards meeting the goal, e.g. a walk every day, being more assertive in a work situation, and to use the hot flush diary to record and monitor specific activities. Suggest daily relaxation practice in a quiet room at a specified time which can be noted on the daily diary with an X plus using paced breathing at onset of hot flushes and if waking during the night. (5 mins)
- Debrief discussion of any questions. (5 mins)

Having this summary near to hand during the session can help with timing.

SESSION 2

The second session focuses on reducing stress and enhancing wellbeing. This is an integral part of the intervention given the impact of stress on hot flushes, as well as quality of life.

Group members may have multiple stressors and responsibilities, and of course stress is a normal part of life. Common sources of stress include: work, health, relationship difficulties, responsibilities for children, grandchildren and/or elderly relatives. Despite their experience of breast cancer, women within the breast cancer groups often report that once their active treatment (radiotherapy, chemotherapy and/or surgery) has finished, they may be expected (by themselves and/or by others) to 'get back to normal' and resume responsibilities that had been put on hold, regardless of the continuing impact of treatment on their energy levels. As a consequence, they may neglect their own emotional and physical needs and put the needs of others and external demands first.

The main aim of this session is therefore to promote the importance of managing stressful situations and to facilitate wellbeing. This is achieved by making cognitive and behavioural changes to reduce stress, which can have a significant impact on their hot flushes. Stress is known to impact on the thermo-neutral zone, and reminding participants of the rationale behind the session can provide motivation for them to engage in behaviour change to manage stress. The session also introduces simple cognitive behavioural strategies providing a foundation on which to build in subsequent weeks.

What will you need?

Flip chart and pens
Homework sheets 4–6
Hot flush weekly diaries
A watch or clock

Agenda

Session 2, Slide 1

As in the previous session, the agenda can be displayed and reviewed at the beginning of the session. The facilitator can then add any additional queries or questions and record them for discussion at the end of the session.

Session 2 example agenda

Review homework – Identifying and modifying precipitants
Stress management and improving wellbeing
Setting individual wellbeing goals
Relaxation and paced breathing
Homework setting

REVIEW HOMEWORK – LOOK AT DIARIES AND DISCUSS PRECIPITANTS OF HOT FLUSHES. ENCOURAGE GROUP MEMBERS TO CONSIDER LIFESTYLE CHANGES TO MODIFY PRECIPITANTS

Feedback on the past week's homework: Look at diaries and discuss precipitants and their relationships to hot flushes.

Session 2, Slide 2

At the end of the first session, group members were asked to look out for and record any precipitants to hot flushes that they may have noticed during the week. Using the flip chart from last week, participants are asked to discuss as a group, any new precipitants to be added to the list. It is not uncommon for participants to feedback that they did not identify any precipitants. In this situation, the facilitator can normalise this, reminding them that studies have shown up to 50 per cent of hot flushes do not have an identifiable precipitant.

Group members are encouraged to find ways to modify precipitants. They can then begin to exercise an element of control over their hot flushes by identifying and modifying trigger situations. Participants can do this by working in pairs and selecting a precipitant that they would like to modify. The facilitator can record the suggestions (e.g. reduce caffeine, cut down alcohol consumption, don't rush, practise breathing when stressed) on the flip chart and ask them to implement these as homework for next week. If someone is unsure how to modify their chosen precipitant, the group may be able to contribute suggestions based on what they may have found helpful.

A balance needs to be established between minor modifications to behaviour or environment and 'cooling or safety behaviours'. Opening windows, layering clothes for easy removal and the use of paced breathing can be helpful strategies and therefore should be encouraged. While safety behaviours, such as avoiding situations, leaving situations, or covering one's face are neutral or less helpful. The aim here is to make small changes to identified precipitants that can be taken to reduce the likelihood of a hot flush happening while continuing with daily tasks.

At the end of the discussion each person should have a goal to reduce hot flush triggers that they will try out in the next week and feed back to the group in Session 3. Participants could also try recording hot flushes and night sweats in the daily diary with and without the modification to see if there is an observable difference, i.e. to experiment to see if modification of the trigger works.

STRESS MANAGEMENT, IMPROVING WELLBEING AND HEALTHY LIFESTYLE (HANDOUTS 4–6)

The main part of the second session is on managing stress, given that stress is believed to further narrow the thermo-neutral zone making women more prone to hot flushes. It is a longer section and the facilitator spends time explaining concepts and including examples from group members. Women then have time to plan an individualised stress-reducing goal for themselves. Focusing on enhancing wellbeing, as well as talking about reducing stress, highlights the importance of looking after oneself and developing a healthy lifestyle. Participants may be reluctant to, or unfamiliar with, putting their own needs first so the facilitator may ask them to think about the potential advantages of reducing stress, for example, improving their ability to manage unavoidable stress when it arises, as is the case for everyone.

For some people prioritising their own needs not only requires a change in their behaviour but also an important shift in the way they think about, and value, themselves in relation to others. From our experience, participants who achieve this cognitive shift at the beginning lay positive foundations for the way they approach the rest of the course. They tend to report a positive impact on wellbeing at the following session, which then motivates them to maintain the changes and to continue to make further positive changes. The group is often a vital vehicle in this change, particularly with cognitive change and therefore getting feedback from each participant prior to the end of the session, especially if they are struggling, opens up the opportunity for other group members to offer support and suggestions.

Sample introductory text

So you'll remember last week that we looked at a cognitive behavioural model of hot flushes and some of the factors that can influence hot flushes, in addition to changes in hormone levels. Today we are going to start looking at one of these factors by looking at lifestyle and stress and ways to facilitate wellbeing. We will start by finding out about stress and then look at ways that we can improve wellbeing by reducing stress. We will also talk about looking after ourselves and managing fatigue and tiredness. It can be helpful to remember that taking care of yourself doesn't mean becoming selfish. Taking care of yourself and looking after your needs enables you to participate more fully in all aspects of life. For a start it will help you to feel more relaxed and have more energy to deal with stressful situations when they arise. We will look at problem solving as well as setting up more positive and rewarding activities.

The session also really reinforces the shift to a self-management approach and the facilitator can highlight this in terms of thinking about investment and benefits.

Stress within the context of the CBT model

Session 2, Slide 3

Following the introduction, the facilitator briefly revisits the CBT model, highlighting the stress and lifestyle section as the part of the model that will be addressed. The facilitator can then summarise the content prior to beginning the section:

- Psycho-education about stress
- The physiology of stress: recognising the signs
- A cognitive behavioural model of stress
- Managing stress and facilitating wellbeing.

Psycho-education – What is stress?

Session 2, Slide 4

The facilitator normalises stress as part of everyday life and explains the important role of cognition or perspective in the experience of stress: stress occurs when environmental, physical, emotional or intellectual demands are placed on somebody. The events or demands are stressful when an individual views the demands as too great and/or evaluates themselves as being unable to meet these demands or unable to cope. This definition of stress explains individual differences in reaction to situations and is a good introduction to the influence of thinking on emotion.

For example, a hectic day may lead person A to rush from one event to another. Person A may then start to *think* that they can't make it on time to the next meeting or arrangement, and they won't possibly be able to fit everything in and get everything done. They evaluate themselves negatively and focus on potential negative consequences (e.g. people will be angry with them, or they will lose their job). This would result in them feeling more stressed. Person B may have the same busy day, which places the same demands on them as they rush from one event to another. Person B however thinks that they will generally manage to fit everything in, and if they are stuck for time, they may have to reschedule something. They may think about the unrealistic nature of the demands and external factors, such as tricky situations at work, concluding that they can't be everywhere at once. Person B is less likely to feel stressed because of their different evaluation of the situation, which enables them to consider several factors that may be contributing to it.

Stress is caused by the perceived *demand of the situation* as well as the individual's negative predictions of whether they will be able to meet these demands (Slide 4). The group can then brainstorm things that they find stressful currently which can be recorded on a flip chart. It is useful for them to use current examples as these can be discussed during the session and then implemented as homework. The facilitator must emphasise that the session is about everyday situations rather than major life events and that the stress management strategies are aimed at everyday stressors.

If someone brings a major life event to the discussion, it can be helpful for the facilitator to offer to discuss this at the end of the session and bring the group back to task. The potential for this can be identified at assessment by including a check on potential major stressors prior to starting the group. The facilitator may then be able to refer the person on to relevant support, or clinical service, if appropriate. Ideally any major stress that might impact on group participation would have already been discussed at the assessment session and a decision made as to whether the person is suitable for the Group CBT or whether she might best have alternative help first. In our experience, with the right preparation, most women are able to find a current stress that it can be beneficial to work on.

The physiology of stress: recognising the signs

Session 2, Slide 5

Once group members have identified a stressful situation, the facilitator explains the physiology of stress, or the 'fight or flight' response, and how people typically experience these physiological responses in their bodies. Participants may be familiar with aspects of the fight or flight response and so the facilitator can first get an idea of participants' understandings by asking them what they think are the main bodily reactions when people are stressed before they explain the physiology of stress.

Sample explanation of physiological aspects of stress

Our ancestors faced real threats and dangers, such as predators, which our bodies are designed to respond to quickly in order to save our lives. This lifesaving response still exists today but is no longer as important given the safety of modern life. When faced with danger, our bodies respond by releasing adrenaline to prepare to fight the danger or run away as quickly as possible. Several things may happen to our bodies, such as the heart beats faster to make sure that the blood is pumped round the body quickly to supply the muscles with enough oxygen and energy to mobilise your body into action – this can be experienced as palpitations. Our breathing becomes faster and deeper to enable the lungs to take in more oxygen for imminent action – this can also lead to dizziness and light-headedness. Our muscles tense to help the body to fight or run. However, ongoing tension may also lead to headaches, indigestion and 'butterflies', shakiness and sweating to help the body to keep cool while running away. In the twenty-first century other kinds of stresses, such as work deadlines, being late, and family responsibilities lead our bodies to react in the same way. Our bodies are unable to distinguish between life-threatening danger and other modern day stresses, so they tend to respond in the same way, which can lead to symptoms of stress and anxiety.

A cognitive behavioural model of stress

Session 2, Slide 6

Next the group can be asked to give examples of their own typical bodily reactions that occur during their stressful situation – these can then be linked into the broader cognitive and behavioural symptoms of stress. The facilitator can then highlight the physical, cognitive, behavioural and emotional components of stress, i.e. how we tend to think, behave and feel a certain way when we are under pressure, drawing on examples provided by the group. In particular, stressful thinking should be a focus using the 'stressful situation' examples participants suggested earlier to draw out specific cognitions about situations. Using a ready prepared flip chart with the cognitive behavioural model presented in the first session drawn on it, participants' answers can be recorded in the relevant box. This can help them to start to separate thoughts and feelings so it is helpful for the facilitator to label suggestions verbally before writing them down or alternatively ask the group to suggest where they go in the diagram.

To help participants differentiate between different components which commonly cause confusion, in particular emotions versus physical feelings, thoughts versus behaviours, it can be useful to draw a smiley or sad face next to the emotions box, and introduce the concept of thought 'bubbles' similar to a comic strip character for thinking. For behaviours, they can be asked to consider what they are 'doing' and maybe adding this in brackets to the diagram.

Example of drawing out cognitive behavioural stress responses

'So when you were asked to finish the project at work by Friday, you thought to yourself "I'm never going to get this done!" (Facilitator records under 'thoughts' part of diagram). How did you feel then?' (Facilitator records 'stressed, worried . . .' under 'feelings' part of diagram and palpitations and tension etc. under the physical reactions part or asks the group to distinguish between which bits go where.) 'What did you do then?' (Facilitator records behaviours in the behaviours box.)

It is useful to have a ready-made example or one of the situations that someone has already suggested to help start the group off. The following example can be used if time is short and the facilitator can encourage the group to generate answers such as 'How might this person feel? What might they be thinking?'

Prepared example: A situation at work where there is a deadline to meet

Person A may find this situation stressful as they tell themselves that they *don't* possibly have the time and they'll '*never* get it finished' (thoughts). If they don't finish it, they tell themselves that 'some sort of *disaster* will happen' e.g. 'I'll lose my job or miss out on promotion' (thoughts). As a consequence, they may procrastinate and avoid starting the task in the first place (behaviour), start drinking or smoking (behaviours) to manage their stress. They may *feel* overwhelmed and angry (feelings) at being put in the position in the first place. And they may experience physical symptoms of stress such as tension and headaches, nausea and insomnia (physical reactions).

Person B may have the same deadline, but tell themselves that they 'will get it finished at some point' and 'it's not the end of the world if it's a bit late' (thoughts). They then feel calm and able to cope with the task (feelings) and will get started on it as soon as possible (behaviour).

Session 2, Slide 7

At the end of the exercise, the facilitator should then review this with the group to highlight stressful thinking and how *predictions/cognitions* about the outcome of the situation (i.e. catastrophe) will also have an impact on their level of stress, behaviour and emotions. The facilitator can then present Slide 7 as a summary.

MANAGING STRESS AND IMPROVING WELLBEING

Session 2, Slide 8

Next the facilitator presents a brief outline of strategies to reduce stress and promote wellbeing. The following cognitive and behavioural strategies are included: calmer thinking; pleasant and calming activities (activity scheduling); exercise; pacing activities; problem-solving; positive psychology. These are summarised on the session Handouts 4 and 5. The aim is to generate individual stress management goals appropriate to their own situation and to implement these as homework the following week.

Calm thinking

Because of the complexity of cognitive work, it may take more time to educate participants in these strategies compared with others in the session. It is worth investing time in this section as often changes in cognition precede changes in behaviour and result in a reduction in stress or anxiety. While it may not be possible for participants to identify and challenge stressful or anxious thinking within a week, they usually develop a basic understanding of anxious thinking and start to recognise it, which can be therapeutic.

Cognitive work can be particularly helpful for people with self-critical thinking patterns as it helps them to identify critical self-talk (e.g. 'Hurry up!' or 'That's awful! What am I doing?') that can lead to increased stress in an already stressful situation, and to develop a more self-supportive, accepting approach to daily pressures. By recognising the pressure placed upon themselves, group members are often able to reduce this simply by recognising it as anxious or stressful thinking. They are then able to take a calmer approach to daily tasks (behaviour change).

Session 2, Slide 9

For the purposes of the intervention, a brief strategy is used to help participants to identify anxious thinking and generate alternative and more self-supportive perspectives. To illustrate this approach, using the flip chart, the facilitator can pick an example presented by one or more group members and run through a number of brief questions to generate a calmer, self supportive alternative thought in the stressful situation. It is important for the facilitator to emphasise that identifying thoughts takes practice but becomes easier with time. Again, asking them to think about the contents of a 'thought bubble' in that situation can help facilitate understanding in the majority of participants. Alternatively, asking participants what they *worried would happen in the situation may give rise to anxious thinking*. Once the thought is identified, the participant may then be asked to rate their stress level out of 10. The facilitator can then work systematically through a series of brief questions to try and generate an alternative self-supportive thought within the situation. This information is included on Handout 4 for group members to take home.

Q: What are the advantages and disadvantages of thinking in this way?
Participants often come up with numerous disadvantages, such as '*I feel worried or stressed'; 'I end up shouting at the children'; 'I work later than I normally would and become tired.*' They are also likely to struggle to generate advantages. Occasionally they may find that stress helps them to get things done. This is fine as long as they are able to recognise the negative impact of self-critical or anxious thinking on their emotions, behaviour and physical wellbeing.

Q: If a friend was feeling stressed and telling themselves [anxious thought], would you agree with them 100 per cent? If not, what would you say to your friend?
This question can help participants to take a step back and consider their current approach from a different perspective. Using the previous example about work pressures, the facilitator may ask, 'Would you agree 100 per cent and tell your friend "*You'll never get the task finished and you'll lose your job*"?' The idea of predicting disaster to an anxious friend often amuses the group and stated so starkly, often helps people to realise the overly negative nature of the thought, and generate a moderate alternative. The facilitator can then record the alternative perspective on a flip chart.

Q: Would a friend see the situation differently? Would they agree with this way of thinking or would they have a different view on this?
It can be helpful for the facilitator to repeat the thought to the group and ask them to consider if a trusted friend would agree with their thinking. Participants may be asked to consider a friend or family member who is generally laid back and calm and ask them to imagine what that person may think of the situation, and what they may advise them to do. It is likely that their calm friend or family member may offer an alternative perspective of the situation. The facilitator can then record the alternative perspective.

Using the answers to the questions above, group members can consider a calmer approach to support themselves within the situation. Once this has been generated, the group can then be asked to re-rate their stress level out of 10 to illustrate the link between thinking and emotions.

Case example

Sue's stressful situation was pressure at work. She felt unable to say no to tasks, constantly had colleagues knocking on her door, and often ended up doing things for others, as this was 'easier and quicker' in the long run. This resulted in her feeling overwhelmed and irritable (emotional consequences) at work and she was behind with her workload (behavioural consequences). Sue then felt tired and tense (physiological consequences) at the end of the day. She also reported a high incidence of hot flushes at work (physiological consequences). With help from the group Sue identified that she had difficulty saying no to people and ended up doing things for them because of the thought 'If I don't do this, nobody else will and it will never get done'. Using the thought challenging questions she identified the disadvantages of this cognitive approach as worry and stress (emotions), taking too much on and being unable to say no to people (behaviours). She realised that she was making assumptions without testing them so she had never found out what would happen if she did delegate tasks; her anxious thinking predicted a negative outcome ('it will never get done') so she always stepped in to prevent this from happening. She identified that she would advise a friend in this situation to delegate tasks and trust others would do them. She would also advise a friend to shut the office door for an hour a day to get on with her job. She thought a calm friend would reassure her that 'things would get done by others' and that 'she would never find this out until she delegated tasks to other people'. This change in thinking then led to two stress goals: (i) to delegate certain tasks to others and (ii) to shut her office door for an hour a day using a 'Do Not Disturb' sign. Sue was initially anxious as she 'predicted' that this would cause difficulties with other staff members. However, she reported the following week that others had completed tasks without difficulty, which lightened her workload. Colleagues respected the office door being closed and she had been able to concentrate on doing her own work. She reported feeling calmer and more in control at work, less irritable with others, and, importantly, she also reported a reduction in severe hot flushes at work.

A few points are pertinent when participants work on this exercise either as a group or in pairs:

- The aim of the exercise is not about unrealistic 'overly positive' thinking, it is about generating less anxious and more neutral or supportive thoughts that help the person to cope within the situation. This fits with an overall aim of the group to encourage participants to facilitate self-care and prioritise their needs.
- In the case of self-criticism in particular, it is helpful to highlight the difference between what participants may tell themselves in a situation, and what they may advise a friend. Linking self-critical thinking to emotions helps to illustrate this. A good analogy is to imagine how they would feel if they had somebody following them around all day, criticising everything they do. Even someone in a reasonable mood would feel more negative as the day progresses, whether that is due to frustration or feeling negative about themselves and their ability.
- If the cognition is worry about what others may be thinking, it is helpful for the facilitator to open this out to the group and ask them to generate other things that people may think in that situation. Ask the group to imagine if they asked 100 people what they were thinking, whether they would *all* agree with the perspective, or whether there would be a range of perspectives or ideas about the situation.
- If a group member is really struggling to find an alternative, the groups are usually very supportive in communicating what they thought of the situation and offering alternative views. Receiving warm and positive support from other group members is helpful in addressing negative thinking and also highlighting the different perspectives of others.

Positive psychology

Another cognitive approach is very quick and simple to carry out. It takes up a few minutes each day and involves the participant reflecting back over the day and jotting down three things that they felt grateful for or that went well. These could be small things like the bus turning up on time, somebody being helpful or friendly to them, or even noticing that the weather was nice. The rationale behind this approach is that it helps the mind to develop a more balanced view of the world and not become too pre-occupied with stresses, strains and negative events. Additionally, if group members have not managed to make time to schedule in a pleasant event, thinking about the day and focusing on something positive that has happened and the feelings they experienced can help lift their mood.

Behavioural strategies to manage stress

In addition to the brief cognitive work, participants are also asked to consider a number of behavioural strategies to help them to manage stress. These are drawn from cognitive behavioural approaches for depression, anxiety and chronic fatigue. After the facilitator has presented these to the group, participants can then work in small groups or pairs to identify which cognitive and/or behavioural strategy they will implement as homework. At the end of this section, each group member should have generated and recorded a goal.

Engaging in pleasant activities: Participants can be encouraged to identify activities that help them to feel relaxed or content and then to schedule them in throughout the week in a realistic quantity that they will be able to fit in. Even 15 minutes with a magazine and a cup of tea can provide a little bit of time out of their day to switch off and can help them to feel more positive about themselves. They are encouraged to set specific measurable goals (e.g. reading for 20 minutes per day) as their homework; these will be reviewed with the group the following week. In addition, if activities are identified that lead to participants feeling drained, stressed or deflated these should be examined and questioned as to whether they are essential or whether alternatives could be adopted, e.g. binge eating, picking an argument. Group discussion in pairs or as a whole group can help to encourage these activities.

Engaging in some exercise: Alongside pleasant activities, physical activity has been found to have a positive effect on both psychological and physical wellbeing and can also help to increase energy levels and improve sleep. It is recommended as a treatment for mild to moderate depression. Therefore exercise in any form is an important activity for participants to engage in, particularly given the prevalence of sleep difficulties, low mood and fatigue in this population. The menopause literature gives conflicting evidence in terms of the impact of exercise on hot flushes. While vigorous exercise can induce a hot flush, overall those who engage in moderate exercise, such as brisk walks, swimming, walking upstairs, report fewer hot flushes. Exercise is also beneficial for mood and sleep. Additionally participants can do activities with friends to introduce a social element to the activity. They may recognise that, while activities such as swimming or walking their dog help them to wind down, they are often the first activities to stop if they feel stressed. The facilitator can emphasise that exercising can lessen the physiological impact of stress and maintain a feeling of wellbeing during

Sample introduction to pleasant activities

Engaging in pleasant activities and taking time for yourself also helps to improve mood. If you are tired or low in mood, you may feel more lethargic by doing nothing. Your mind is also not occupied so you are more likely to brood about problems or difficulties you may be having and feel even worse. Scheduling in pleasant activities and making time for yourself is rewarding since, at the very least, it can take your mind off things and by investing more time in yourself, you may start to feel more positive and more in control of your life. It can help to rate your mood before and after to see how this works, which I can show you how to do. If you enjoy exercise, then you can combine exercise and scheduling pleasant activities.

Think of things that you used to enjoy or small things that give you pleasure or that are relaxing.

stressful times. As with activity scheduling, a specific goal can be measured and reviewed the following week when the group review homework.

Session 2, Slide 10

Pacing activities: While activity pacing was initially developed as part of interventions for fatigue, it can be a useful strategy for people with numerous responsibilities and busy lives. It is particularly useful for women recovering from breast cancer who may still be feeling fatigue following their treatment regime. The facilitator can explain the impact of all or nothing bouts of activity in terms of the 'boom and bust' cycle and acknowledge the temptation to cram lots of activities in if their energy levels feel higher.

Taking regular breaks, as well as breaking down big tasks into smaller manageable parts with a break in-between, are also important components of pacing. The facilitator should acknowledge the temptation to do more on good days and how this may be frustrating in the short term. However, it should be emphasised that in the long term this can help participants to slowly build up their activity levels without wearing themselves out and eventually get more done as they are less likely to wear themselves out.

Sample pacing description

Pacing is a skill, which helps when you are tired or have a lot on your plate and feel overwhelmed. It helps to maintain reasonable levels of energy without wearing yourself out. Pacing involves not overdoing things on days where you have more energy as this can lead to you feeling overtired, which can make small tasks even more challenging. Therefore it is about reaching a balance so that you consistently do activities at the same pace regardless of whether you are having a good day or a bad day. It is helpful to keep an activity diary over the course of a week measuring how much you can comfortably manage on good days and bad days then average this out. Once you have an average amount of activity, take 10–20 per cent off and use this as your initial daily activity schedule. Although this may feel frustrating at first, you can gradually build this up as your body adapts. If you are able to practise pacing regularly, it may be that you have fewer tired days or are able to accomplish tasks on days when you are tired or low in mood by pacing them and giving yourself breaks. Another aspect of pacing is to break down huge tasks into smaller manageable tasks, that you can complete one at a time with regular breaks. Again, this is more efficient in the long run and avoids a boom and bust cycle of energy.

Problem-solving

Session 2, Slide 11

When a specific situation is causing stress and action is needed to resolve the situation (as opposed to taking a different cognitive perspective or using relaxation), problem-solving is a useful strategy to use. Problem-solving is commonly used in CBT interventions for depression and worry. Slide 11 and Handout 5 show the diagram, which is given to participants and briefly explained. The facilitator can emphasise that problem-solving may not provide a 'perfect solution' but rather will enable them to consider the possible options that are available to address the problem and use calm reasoning to decide which course to take.

Session 2, Slides 12, 13 and 14

Sample problem-solving summary

Identify the problem – *sometimes the most difficult step is identifying the stressor – what is the actual problem? If you are having difficulty, it may help to sit down and chat with someone outside of the situation. If you have a number of different stressors, then these should be separated into individual issues and problem-solving applied to each.*

List all possible solutions – *once you have identified the issues that are stressing you out, make a list of potential options available to you, which would help address the problem. List everything you come up with, even silly suggestions – it may help to list the worst possible thing you can do, as well as the 'ideal' option which may not be possible – the solution will lie somewhere in-between. Discuss it with somebody else and jot down their ideas too. Consider also who may be able to help you out in each solution.*

Consider the pros and cons of each action – *write down the advantages and disadvantages of each solution. Think about the short term and the long term consequences and consider the impact on yourself and others for each solution. Once you have started this process, the list of options should start to reduce into a few good possibilities.*

Identify the best option – *remember this doesn't have to be a perfect solution but one with the most advantages, and fewer disadvantages. Think about ways you can manage the disadvantages.*

Summarising cognitive and behavioural strategies using **Slides 12 and 13** then offers participants a reference point as they work in pairs to identify their stress goals **(Session 2, Slide 14).** Working in pairs offers participants the opportunity to discuss their own situation and gain a different perspective than they might get if working alone. The facilitator can walk around the group offering help if needed while participants discuss and complete the task. If there is time at the end, participants can briefly feed their goal back to the group. It is best if each participant sets a specific goal, which is measurable. So for example rather than 'reading more' or 'do more exercise', it could be that they aim to read for 15–20 minutes per day or 30 minutes of a specific exercise three times per week. This is then easier for them to monitor and feed back.

GROUP RELAXATION EXERCISE, TENSING AND RELAXING MUSCLES THROUGH THE BODY AND FOCUS ON PACED BREATHING

Session 2, Slide 15

Before doing the relaxation, it is useful to get brief feedback about participants' experiences of the relaxation homework that was set the past week. If women were able to practise this, they typically talk about benefits following the relaxation in terms of their energy, improved management of hot flushes and feeling relaxed:

'Concentrating on my breathing when I had a flush did actually stop it . . . [and] stopped me feeling dizzy.'

'Relaxation made me feel energised.'

Participants often report practising the relaxation at different times of the day, for example before going to bed to help them relax and go to sleep, or before work to prepare them for the day ahead. Others practise it whenever they felt stressed during the day. Those who had not managed to practise the relaxation or had only practised it once were often motivated to try it out the following week after listening to positive feedback of other group members. Even so, the facilitator can check for barriers to relaxation and encourage the group to troubleshoot these barriers for the individual who perhaps has not had time. The facilitator's role is to encourage participants to maintain this practice in order to develop the skill further and to eventually enable them to be able to slip into a more relaxed state with less effort as the intervention proceeds.

Introducing paced breathing into relaxation

This week, the focus of the relaxation exercise begins to shift to paced breathing. Descriptions of this vary, but we suggest slow diaphragmatic breathing. Some people suggest counting to five for the inhalation and five again for the exhalation. Participants should be encouraged to adopt whatever is helpful to them and to avoid holding their breath. The main message is simply to find a gentle rhythm and focus their attention on their breathing – if it helps them to count then they should count, if not, as long as they are able to shift their attention to breathing, that is fine. Before and throughout the relaxation, the facilitator can normalise the experience of the mind wandering. Group members can be encouraged to notice that their mind has wandered to other thoughts, and then, without fighting the thought, gently bring their attention back to their breathing and focus on the sensation of air entering and leaving their body.

Sample paced breathing description

Becoming skilled at paced breathing is useful when an uncomfortable or intense symptom arises. At first it may be difficult to remember to become aware of the breath but regular practice is beneficial. It can also help to practise when annoying or irritating experiences occur. For example, if you're waiting in a queue and the person in front is really slow, acknowledge that you're irritated or impatient e.g. 'I feel really annoyed/frustrated' and then follow that by becoming aware of your breath and the breath as it flows in and out of your body. It can help to be quite conscious of the process saying to yourself, 'Breathe in, tummy expanding, breathing out, tummy softening' or something similar. Feel the body letting go with each outward breath. Once you have followed the breath for a minute or so, the situation may have resolved itself and you've had the pleasure of a few minutes of calming breathing. Or if not, you have created space in your mind for how to react calmly. Let shoulders relax at the onset of the flush, breathe slowly from your stomach and concentrate on your breathing. Allow the flush to flow over you as you relax.

Group relaxation exercise: tensing and relaxing muscles through the body and focus on paced breathing for 10 minutes. At the end of this relaxation session, participants are encouraged to practise using the recording as homework for the week and to practise paced breathing if they notice themselves feeling stressed, at the onset of a hot flush, or if woken by a night sweat. The facilitator can remind participants that they will be asked to feed this back next week.

HOMEWORK SUMMARY AND REVIEW

Session 2 Slide 15

The following homework is set for this session:

1. Implement and monitor modifications to hot flush precipitants identified as last week's homework.
2. Introduce cognitive behavioural strategies from wellbeing/stress management plan. (Handout 6)
3. Continue daily relaxation practice including paced breathing.
4. Practise paced breathing at the start of a flush, night sweat or during a stressful situation.

DEBRIEF DISCUSSION OF ANY QUESTIONS, GIVE OUT HANDOUTS AND DIARIES

4

Session 3: Managing hot flushes using a cognitive behavioural approach

SUMMARY OF SESSION 3

- Review homework on identifying and modifying precipitants to hot flushes, as well as stress/wellbeing goals. Look at diaries and discuss precipitants, relaxation practice and relationships to hot flushes. Feed back on wellbeing and stress goals. Discussion of dealing with stress goals, e.g. a walk every day, taking time for oneself for an hour a day. Encourage the use of the diary to record specific activities. (15 mins)
- Dealing with hot flushes – *thoughts and beliefs*. Discussion of thoughts and beliefs about menopause and hot flushes and possible meanings of symptoms in the context of breast cancer. Discuss thoughts that women have before, during and after a hot flush. Write down on flip chart. Discuss other people's reactions to menopausal symptoms and how to deal with social situations. Discuss evidence for and against negative automatic thoughts and assumptions about hot flushes and menopause. Identify strategies for managing these situations using the evidence and brainstorm alternative more helpful thoughts (Handout 7–10). Homework: to be aware of thoughts and assumptions and to write them down. (45 mins)
- Behavioural reactions and strategies to manage hot flushes. Paced breathing linked in as a behavioural strategy. What is helpful or unhelpful. (Handout 11) (15 mins)
- Group relaxation exercise. Shorter form of relaxing muscles through the body and focus on paced breathing. Homework: daily practice in quiet room at specified time plus using *paced breathing at onset of hot flushes* and before going to sleep and if wake up at night. (10 mins)
- Debrief discussion of any questions and summarise homework. Homework: To develop individual cognitive behavioural goals to try out as homework and feed back during the next session. (5 mins)
- At the end of the session:
  Give out sleep diary at the end of the session for women to complete the following week in order to provide information about their sleep pattern for next session.

SESSION 3

Session 3 Slide 1

The third session aims to enable participants to identify thinking patterns and behavioural reactions so that they can make some changes to help them to manage hot flushes and feel more in control. As a consequence, they should be able to reduce distress they may experience when having a hot flush. While the session covers cognitive and behavioural change, the main focus of the session is on cognitive aspects of hot flushes. The reasons for this are twofold: often women are using reasonable behavioural strategies and have already started to use breathing and relaxation during a flush following on from the previous two sessions. Second, behavioural change often involves changes to thinking within situations. Participants often need to identify and examine beliefs about hot flushes in order to make the behavioural changes that facilitate coping. This is evident in the stress case studies in the previous session and will be illustrated in relation to hot flushes specifically later in this chapter.

Have a copy of this summary in the session to keep a check on content and timing.

What will you need?

Flip chart and pens
Handouts 7–12
Hot flush weekly diaries
A watch/clock
CBT worksheet to address hot flush thinking and behaviour
Sleep Diary

Agenda

As in previous sessions, the facilitator can display the agenda at the beginning.

Session 3 example agenda

Review Homework: Precipitant identification and modification
Stress/wellbeing goals and relaxation review
Managing hot flushes by changing thinking
Managing hot flushes by changing behaviour
Relaxation and paced breathing
Homework setting

HOMEWORK REVIEW: IDENTIFYING AND MODIFYING PRECIPITANTS TO HOT FLUSHES, AS WELL AS STRESS/WELLBEING GOALS

Session 3, Slide 2

Homework for Session 2 involved modifying precipitants, continuing to practise relaxation and breathing, as well as implementing goals to reduce stress and enhance their wellbeing. The size of the group and the time constraints will influence how the goals are discussed and fed back. A large group might discuss their progress in pairs and feedback to the group anything that they may have had difficulty with, so that the group can support them in troubleshooting difficulties. Alternatively, if the group is relatively small (up to 6), participants may take turns to feed back their goals and outcomes to the group.

Participants often find that they continue to identify new precipitants using the diary even if they have not consciously tried to do so. Following the session on stress, they are likely to report an increased awareness of cognitive behavioural factors and their emotional impact. Conversely, women also tend to notice the situations in which they did not have hot flushes and then made an effort to spend more time doing these activities. For example, one participant reported that she didn't have any hot flushes when she was gardening and she had therefore started to generally spend more time outside in the garden relaxing or tending the garden.

'I have found gardening very therapeutic, being outside makes me feel better.'

***Mary** recognised that her hot flushes were often triggered if she had an argument or disagreement with her husband. As she recognised that she often started these arguments, particularly after a stressful day at work, she realised that she could choose not to start the argument in the first place and instead had started to take time out to relax and calm down after work. This approach incorporated the homework on modifying precipitants from the previous week, noticing emotional triggers, as well as consciously taking more care of herself, in order to enhance her own wellbeing.*

***Suzie** reported that she had hot flushes when meeting friends in the pub, which initially she was surprised at as she viewed this as a pleasant situation. Specifically, she had noticed the hot flush was triggered when her friends talked about negative situations at work and the conversation became heated. Suzie reported that instead of joining in with the 'fierce discussion', she excused herself at the beginning of this topic and went to the toilet and did some paced breathing. By the time she returned she had been able to think about what she could contribute to the conversation without becoming irate, 'I concentrated on my breathing and thought about what I was going to do next . . .' When she rejoined the conversation she contributed calmly. She had since started focusing her attention on her breathing in similar situations when friends phoned her.*

Discussion of achievements or barriers can draw on group support to reinforce changes and encourage next steps. The homework goals also involved the application of cognitive and behavioural strategies to manage stress and enhance wellbeing, making time for oneself to practise relaxation, and developing an emphasis on self-care and meeting one's own needs. Women are encouraged to continue and set new stress/wellbeing goals. The group gradually becomes familiar with issues that group members are working on and group reinforcement is helpful. Barriers to practice should be accepted and participants are encouraged to find ways to overcome these, with the understanding that any small change is helpful and that people's choices, progress and lifestyles will differ.

***Anna** reported that during the week she had realised at work that she was 'telling myself off all of the time and rushing'. She had found it difficult to identify any stressful thoughts during the session the previous week and expressed surprise that she was being so 'unkind' to herself. At work, she recalled the previous session and remembered the cognitive work about whether a friend would agree with this way of thinking, and whether she would agree with the thought if a friend had it. She generated an alternative calmer approach to work and had found that she was less stressed during the week. She reported that she was, 'Relaxing my attitude . . . I am being my own best friend . . . When I notice this, I talk out loud [and tell myself] "Stop Rushing" . . . I am supporting myself and being positive.'*

***Carmen** reported feeling much less stressed at the beginning of this session. She put this down to her awareness of the role of thinking in exacerbating stress and so was keeping a check on thoughts. She gave an example of having her bike stolen and instead of ruminating about what had happened (engaging with negative thinking)* *and becoming really upset about it, she told herself that she was not going to let it bother her all day. As a result, she carried on as usual: 'I am doing much better in stressful situations, I am taking things much more calmly.'*

Taking the pressure off is a common theme. Participants often report feeling less stressed after making relatively minor changes that combine the cognitive and behavioural stress management strategies as well as developing a self-nurturing approach. They also start to talk about how they were bringing breathing and relaxation into this.

'I've been looking after myself, the [relaxation] CD pops into my head and it helped.'

'Being aware of and avoiding negative thoughts. Breathing helps as well.'

MANAGING HOT FLUSHES USING A COGNITIVE BEHAVIOURAL APPROACH. DEALING WITH HOT FLUSHES – *THOUGHTS AND BELIEFS*

Session 3, Slide 3

Handouts 7 and 8 (Handout 9 is a worksheet summarising the cognitive strategies in detail for participants to take home and read)

This section comprises the main body of the session and builds upon preliminary cognitive and behavioural skills that were introduced in Session 2. The facilitator can mention that the advice is based on research findings that beliefs and thoughts about menopause and about hot flushes can influence individual experience of them and how people cope. S/he should take care to emphasise that hot flushes are distressing, particularly in social situations such as work or in situations in which participants may feel uncomfortable.

First, the facilitator asks the group to do a word association for 'Menopause' and writes the responses on a flip chart. The aim of this is to help group members to develop an awareness of the social meanings of menopause and also the nature of their own automatic thoughts. This is a very quick exercise where group members can shout out words that spring to mind when the menopause is mentioned. Within the groups, answers provided tend to reflect negative connotations of menopause (e.g. 'old', 'past it', 'stressed and bothered', 'unattractive'). After this has been completed, the facilitator can lead a brief discussion of personal meanings of menopause and the socio-cultural context of menopause.

Sample information about meanings of menopause

Menopause is still a relatively taboo topic. The menopause has for centuries been associated with emotional and physical problems, particularly in Western cultures, and negative assumptions about its impact upon sexual function, femininity, ageing and women's mental health are still prevalent in the media today. 'The change' or 'change of life' is a commonly used term reflecting the view that the meaning of the menopause is closely associated with general psychological and social adaptations of midlife. Physical and psychological experiences or symptoms that are often attributed to the menopause in Western cultures include hot flushes, night sweats, irregular and/or heavy periods, but also depression, headaches, insomnia, anxiety and weight gain. However, apart from menstrual changes, hot flushes and night sweats, and also vaginal dryness, are the only 'symptoms' that have been found to be clearly associated with the menopause and changes in hormone levels.

Media portrayals of women and medical writings about menopause in the Western world have contributed to a stereotypically negative picture of the menopausal woman as irritable, depressed, asexual and besieged by hot flushes. Oestrogen therapy was prescribed for flushes and night sweats initially, in the 1940s in the USA when menopause was seen as an 'oestrogen deficiency disease', a cluster of physical and emotional symptoms that should be 'treated', rather than a normal phase of women's lives. The promotion of oestrogen therapy focused on a range of negative consequences of the menopause, the message being that if you didn't treat the menopause you will be unattractive and unhealthy and in a state of decline! Furthermore, in many cultures, women tend to be valued for their physical and sexual attractiveness, reproductive capacity and youthfulness. Negative attitudes to ageing are very common. The focus on 'treatment' of menopause and 'staying young' can be anxiety provoking. There is some evidence that negative attitudes towards menopause can affect symptom experience – a self-fulfilling prophecy. Not too surprising perhaps since if we think that we are going to become 'unattractive, over emotional and prone to long-term illness' this might well affect how we feel. What do you think about menopause? Let's brainstorm the word menopause to find out.

Next the facilitator invites the group to discuss this information and think about how it might influence their experience of hot flushes. The message being that it is not surprising that women often have negative cognitive reactions to their hot flushes, given how menopause tends to be viewed in Western cultures. It is also important to discuss how the women's personal views may be related to their life experience (e.g. their mother's view of menopause and how this was communicated), as well as negative social stereotypes (e.g. how menopausal women are portrayed on the television). To illustrate the latter, ask the women to imagine if menopause was portrayed as a positive life stage for women and was associated with wisdom and increased status, would they feel the same level of negativity towards their hot flushes and menopausal status?

The facilitator introduces the CBT work by reminding participants of how stressful thinking can make difficult situations worse. This session will focus on developing calmer cognitive responses to hot flushes. By doing so, the group can support themselves when having hot flushes using calm and supportive talk, rather than catastrophising and feeling even more anxious or distressed. This helps to develop a more accepting approach to hot flushes, which can reduce distress and improve coping.

Session 3, Slide 4

The facilitator invites the group to either brainstorm cognitive, behavioural and emotional aspects of a hot flush and write them on the flip chart, or discuss their cognitive, emotional and behavioural reactions during a hot flush in pairs and then feed back. The facilitator can lead the discussion and his/her co-facilitator can write down on the flip chart (as in Slide 5).

Sample introduction to cognitive behavioural work

Today we will be covering cognitive aspects of the model, so thoughts and beliefs about the menopause and hot flushes, as well as emotional and behavioural reactions to hot flushes. As we learnt last week, often our thoughts can influence the way we feel and behave in certain situations. In stressful situations such as at work or if you are having a hot flush, these thoughts can make you feel much worse and result in a range of emotions and behaviours. These thoughts are automatic and quick and can be difficult to identify. They may stem from beliefs about menopause that we may take for granted. Because of this we often assume they are right and do not think about them in great detail. Today we are going to look closely at these thoughts, and how they influence feelings and behaviour during a hot flush. We will then examine their helpfulness and see if we can come up with any alternative calmer ways of responding to hot flushes that helps us to cope better when they come along when you least want them to.

We are going to have a look at what happens when you have a hot flush. As a group or in pairs I want you to have a chat about what your experiences are when you have a hot flush. What sort of thoughts go through your head, what do you tell yourself will happen or is happening, how do you feel emotionally and physically, and what you do to cope either during or after a hot flush.

Session 3, Slide 5

Slide 5 has examples suggested by women during group exercises. Often, thoughts arise about feeling out of control due to the frequency or severity of flushes, or are socially anxious in content with participants making assumptions about what other people may think about them during a hot flush.

An important part of the exercise is trying to identify the thought in the first place. Therefore it is worth checking at this point if anyone is struggling to identify their 'hot thoughts'. The facilitator can help to prompt participants by asking them about the last time they had a moderate or severe hot flush:

- *What ran through your head when you realised you were having a hot flush?*
- *What did you tell yourself/think would happen?*
- *Why did you feel particularly frustrated/embarrassed/angry/horrified?*
- *Did you have any images in your head about what may happen?*
- *What do you think other people in the situation may have been thinking?*

Once the brainstorm is complete, the facilitator can use the examples given to remind participants about the nature of stressful thinking. This involves acknowledging the discomfort of the hot flush while also reminding participants that stressful and negative thinking tends to predict a bad outcome and lead to assumptions that they will not be able to cope. A sample explanation is outlined below and Slide 5 is likely to be similar to the group examples identified on the flip chart.

Sample explanation

So from the examples it is clear that people react to hot flushes in different ways in terms of how they think. If you look at the thoughts, you may notice that they are similar to the anxious thoughts or negative automatic thoughts that we identified last week during the stress session. Therefore, while the hot flush is itself distressing, thinking patterns within the situation are often overly negative resulting in feeling even worse. The thoughts exacerbate negative feelings, such as feeling out of control, frustrated and embarrassed, and influence behaviour in the situation. Some of these behaviours may be helpful, such as opening the window to cool down or removing layers, while some may be less helpful such as starting to avoid situations. It is when we start to avoid certain situations that our anxiety about having a hot flush can get bigger still. By recognising and identifying these ways of thinking we can question them and try and generate some helpful alternatives, so that you feel less extreme emotions when having a hot flush, which should help you to feel more in control and coping better.

There is a fine balance between introducing participants to the role of thoughts and behaviours, and acknowledging that hot flushes are a stressful experience, especially in social situations and with people they may not know. The key is to be empathic whilst familiarising them with the impact of catastrophic responses on their feelings and coping strategies. It may be useful for the facilitator to frame the rationale as being about identifying understandable anxious thinking that arises during a hot flush and looking at ways they can 'look after' or 'support' themselves during these times by developing more helpful and calmer thinking. Acknowledging the discomfort whilst also helping women to identify calmer and self-supportive alternatives (e.g. this will be over soon, it won't last forever; other people will be less aware of my hot flushes than I am) is key to engaging the group in the cognitive work.

Occasionally there may be a group participant who does not have catastrophic or anxious thinking about their hot flushes and may have developed a more accepting attitude. This can be helpful to illustrate the cognitive behavioural model to other women when considering alternatives to catastrophic thinking and the subsequent reduction in negative emotions. An example from the groups was:

'It happens to everyone . . . It's just the life stage I'm at, you'll get it at some point [to facilitator].'

This participant did not experience anxiety and tended to engage in calm behaviour. Despite not having any catastrophic thoughts or related negative emotions, this participant fed back to the group that the exercise had enabled her to see she was managing her hot flushes well, and this in turn had built her confidence and helped her to feel more positive about herself.

Session 3, Slides 6 and 7

A number of studies have shown that women's main concerns are in relation to *social embarrassment* and *control*. The facilitator may want to emphasise that everybody will be different and, for example while some women feel they can handle social situations and do not feel embarrassed, for others, these will be the most difficult situations when having a hot flush. In summary, high levels of distress are associated with the following thinking patterns or errors:

- a tendency to catastrophise,
- the use of negative shaming labels,
- higher levels of self-criticism, and

- higher levels of symptom reporting (which may be due to attentional focus on flushes and bodily changes).

Typically, distressed women are unlikely to tell others that they are experiencing hot flushes due to their feelings of shame and therefore their assumptions about a negative reaction go unchallenged. The important message here is not for everyone to necessarily disclose their hot flushes to all and sundry, but rather how the behaviour of the distressed women can reinforce their beliefs about a negative reaction.

The facilitator's role is to guide women to solutions, while enabling them to work together to develop calmer thinking. The message for women therefore is to support themselves during the hot flush, as they would do for others. This can be compared with the stress work in the case of women who may have started developing 'calm self talk' during their daily life (e.g. '*Take your time, there's no rush*').

Social situations

Session 3, Slides 8 and 9

Worries about appearance in front of others can lead women to apply self-critical and highly negative labels ('disgusting', 'unattractive' are common examples), while heightening self-focus and leading to the 'observer perspective'. Consistent with the social anxiety CBT model, these women's views of themselves appear to be derived from internal information such as bodily sensations, emotions arising from the initial cognitive reactions to the hot flush, and a negative judgement on performance within the situation. This then can perpetuate anxiety/embarrassment/shame and potentially hot flush symptoms. Women experiencing these kinds of thoughts tend to have an overly negative self-image, with high expectations of themselves and high levels of self-criticism. Hot flushes might be considered to reduce their ability to meet their high standards. They might then 'define' themselves solely by the hot flush within that situation and ignore all other factors in the situation and other personal qualities they may have. This is illustrated in the following example:

Liz *reported that her hot flushes were most problematic in her work as a lawyer. She would feel one starting and focus her attention on how this develops, reporting that she looked 'disgusting' due to perspiration and she needed to dab her face. Her key cognitions within the situation were 'Everybody will think I'm disgusting' and 'They'll think I'm incompetent'. Subsequently she became very anxious and would often request a break and reschedule the rest of the session by telephone. During this time, nobody had ever commented on her appearance or given any impression they had noticed her symptoms. Liz assumed that her perspiration was not only noticed by everyone but also evaluated negatively, resulting in self-critical thinking and avoidance of the situation whenever possible. Cognitive work within the session focused on identifying thinking errors such as 'mind reading', how she would respond to a client in that situation, and asking Liz to consider other factors that were important within the situation, such as her past relationships with the people involved and her hard work and competence.*

The facilitator should aim to draw women's attention to the potential contribution of cognitive biases in terms of making assumptions about what others may be thinking, without evidence to support their assumptions (mind-reading) (Slide 8). The possible influences of negative stereotypes about menopause (both their own and society's), and the role of the *observer perspective* in increasing self-consciousness and biasing their interpretation of the situation are pointed out. A number of strategies are suggested then to address each issue (Slide 9).

The facilitator can ask women to put themselves in the other person's position and think about the interaction in the context of a few questions. If they are having negative or self critical thoughts, ask them to consider how they might think about someone else having a hot flush, would they:

- Feel negatively towards the person who is perspiring and red?
- Forget everything else you know about them/the purpose of the interaction and be completely pre-occupied about the hot flush?
- Be totally pre-occupied by this for the rest of the day?

These questions should help to begin to draw out a more balanced perspective within the situation by highlighting other factors within the situation and the role of self-criticism.

Other people's views of menopausal symptoms: the survey (summarised in Handout 10)

To provide practical evidence about other people's views we carried out a survey of men and non-menopausal women about their perceptions of menopausal symptoms (Smith et al. 2011). This was done via an anonymous Internet survey targeting working men and non-menopausal women below the age of forty. The results were illuminating and provide evidence that younger men and women have a broad range of attributions regarding hot flush symptoms, and tended to interpret an interaction with a flushed and perspiring colleague in a neutral way. It is helpful to present the results to give women the chance to begin to generate their own alternatives and examine their thoughts closely. The detailed findings can be found in Handout 10, but in summary:

- Younger men and women had a variety of ideas about the possible causes of the redness and perspiration in mid aged women, none of which were overly negative in the way the women had assumed. These included: exercise, embarrassment, stress, room too hot, she may be coming down with a cold.
- Respondents did not report negative reactions, such as disgust or horror at the symptoms. They reported feeling either nothing or some concern about their colleague if they knew them well.
- Respondents were thinking about the appropriateness of *their own* response in the interaction rather than focusing on their colleague's hot flush.
- This evidence is helpful in highlighting some of the cognitive biases discussed by the facilitator, particularly when women struggle to generate alternative views within the situation.

'We're assuming people think the same as us because of our own worry, when others don't actually care . . . They may not notice, they won't care if they do, or they may feel concerned.'

For some, this change in perspective results in a change in behaviour. In the following weeks, women often report that they are more able to comment or joke about a hot flush if they started to have one in a work or social situation. Women typically tend to become less anxious and feel more able to explain their symptoms without feeling ashamed. They often receive positive reactions and/or support from people that they previously would not have expected, for example men might share that their partner/wife was going through similar experience, or women of a similar age might share their own experiences. This further reduces anxiety about having a hot flush in a social situation with people they are less familiar with.

Example of finding helpful alternative thoughts in social situations

Thought: *They will think something is wrong with me (e.g. I'm having a heart attack, or I have a serious physical defect).*
Feelings: *Embarrassment 60 per cent; Uncomfortable 80 per cent.*
Advantages of thinking in this way: *None.*
Disadvantages of thinking this way: *Makes me feel embarrassed, and frustrated.*

Would a friend agree with the anxious thought in this situation?
A friend would probably say that they would be concerned about me, they may not even notice, they will not give the same level of importance to it as I do – they won't really care either way.

What would you say to a friend?
I would tell her that people may not notice most of the time, everybody gets sweaty sometimes, and that menopause is normal and happens to all women. It's none of their business. It will pass and it doesn't matter.

Alternative thoughts:
I am ignoring everything else about the situation and focusing in on one aspect of it which doesn't really matter and it will pass. Every woman goes through it. They probably won't even notice.
Embarrassment: 40 per cent; Uncomfortable 40 per cent.

Control cognitions

Session 3, Slides 10 and 11

The other main types of thoughts are related to the perception of being unable to *control* the flushes. For these cognitions, women tend to report feelings of frustration or irritation about the flush, as well as feeling overwhelmed or helpless. For example, they may feel more able to tolerate flushes when they are mild to moderate, if they are perceived to have an acceptable temporal gap between them, or if there is a clear trigger. However, where the occurrence of the flush violates these 'rules', for example by increasing in severity, running in quick succession, or occurring in a situation where the participant would not expect them (when relaxed, or independently of any identifiable triggers), the participant's thinking can become overly negative.

Common thinking patterns in relation to control include catastrophising (e.g. 'these will *never* end') and applying 'shoulds and oughts', e.g. 'I *shouldn't* be having another one so soon' or 'I *should* be able to control them all the time'. For some women, hot flushes are accompanied by symptoms such as dizziness and nausea. In these cases, participants might report cognitions that can occur during panic attacks (e.g. 'I will pass out/lose control'), which can be helped using cognitive strategies that are effective for people with panic attacks (see page 7).

Lack of control can sometimes stem from women's feelings about the menopause in general. For example, a woman might report her body was 'working against her' in some way, adding to feelings of frustration. The psycho-education on the physiology of hot flushes in the first session can help to normalise the menopause, which in turn can help them to respond more neutrally.

To highlight the role of attention on hot flush sensations, the facilitator can do a brief attention task with women during the session. This is optional but is applicable to social situations where women turn their attention on themselves and general situations where they focus their attention on the hot flush sensations as they are happening. Asking the participants to pick a part of their body and focus on it intensely for 1–2 minutes, looking out for sensations demonstrates the role of hyper-vigilance in intensifying sensations. If women focus on their hands or feet, they tend to report they notice how heavy they are, they notice their pulse or they report feelings of heat. Focusing on the head has similar results although this can be particularly powerful as it can lead to reddening and the start of a build-up of heat. This provides motivation for women to practise shifting their attention outwards or to their breath during a hot flush.

In order to help women tackle these cognitions around control, the facilitator will need to reinforce the natural process their bodies are going through and address assumptions about the 'rules' of hot flushes, as well as linking thoughts to the stress work from last week. This can be done by acknowledging their distress in the situation in terms of the discomfort of the hot flush, while reinforcing the idea that stressful thinking is likely to increase feelings of distress, and potentially the intensity of the flush. A number of strategies can be used:

- Examine the advantages and disadvantages of these types of thoughts by asking women to consider the impact of the thought on the vicious cycle, and in particular their feelings.
- The facilitator can ask the group to consider what a friend might say if they know that they are feeling 'out of control' during a hot flush. This can help to motivate women to consider alternative, more supportive and calming thoughts.
- In terms of anger and frustration, the facilitator can point out that women have a choice about how to respond and can pause and take a breath before they get angry. This is similar to cognitive work for anger; they can either go with their angry thoughts and frustration which then has physiological consequences that may exacerbate the flush, or they can opt for slow breathing and a self supportive statement: 'Stay calm, this will pass', for example. Acknowledging their frustration as normal is an important part of motivating women to try out this strategy. Also encouraging women to try out *both* strategies (going with their frustration versus using calming thinking and behaviour) in the week as homework and to feed back next week any differences they noticed presents this strategy as a behavioural experiment rather than a prescriptive approach. The behavioural experiment approach is particularly helpful in terms of actively comparing strategies.
- Reminding women of the impact of paced breathing can also help to challenge thoughts about not having any control. Additionally asking women to consider other factors that they have discovered so far which have an impact and how they have made changes to manage these. Is the thought 'I am out of control' 100 per cent true in all situations all of the time?
- For some women, flushes are accompanied by nausea and/or dizziness, and fear that they might pass out or collapse. This can then lead to feelings of anxiety and behavioural avoidance of certain situations. To address these worries, women are reminded of the body's response to anxiety provoking situations and how nausea and dizziness can be part of this. Therefore although the symptoms are

uncomfortable, they will not lead to the feared catastrophe of collapse or fainting. This is because bodies are 'activated' (e.g. the heart is pumping, oxygen is flowing) whereas fainting and collapsing are normally preceded by some sort of 'deactivation' (e.g. blood pressure drops, oxygen levels have dropped). In addition women should be encouraged to do paced breathing, which can reduce feelings of dizziness and nausea.

- Checking expectations can help participants to identify the source of frustration. This is helpful for those who experience a series of consecutive flushes (assumption 'There should be a reasonable time gap between flushes') or who cannot identify trigger (assumption 'flushes will never happen when I am relaxed'). Participants will need to be reminded that while 50 per cent are likely to have an identifiable trigger, some will just occur. Therefore, the work within the groups can help to reduce them but not necessarily eradicate them completely.

Example

Sarah reported particularly troublesome flushes following a family weekend during Session 3. She said that she was able to manage flushes at work without a problem using humour with colleagues and opening windows, but at the weekend she had a particularly difficult time when she was relaxing and spending time with her extended family. When this was explored, there was no difference between the number of flushes at work compared with at home but she reported that the flushes at home had been particularly intense. Sarah identified that when she has a hot flush at work, she accepts them as she works in a busy and stressful environment and therefore expects them to happen due to stress being a trigger. Her cognitive response therefore is 'I'm having a hot flush because I am a bit stressed and it will pass in a minute'. Consequently she accepts the flush and copes by focusing her attention on the task she is doing or by making a comment to colleagues before 'just getting on with things' (behaviour). She reported that she doesn't really take much notice of them and they do not cause her distress at work.

At home, in a situation where she feels relaxed and happy, her cognitive response changes. The important difference between the two situations is her ***expectation****. Therefore, when a hot flush occurs, her cognitive response is 'This should not be happening, I am relaxed'. She then feels frustrated and becomes preoccupied with the flushes and the physical sensations, thinking about how they are 'ruining my family time'. Her frustration and anger increase and she spends the afternoon focusing on how many hot flushes she is having. Her frustration was acknowledged but the facilitator noted how the hot flushes were the same, but the situation subsequently impacted on her expectations, which were the root of the distress. Sarah was encouraged to practise the acceptance she was implementing very effectively at work using calming cognitive responses ('this will pass soon'), in addition to paced breathing in order to manage situations at home.*

Additional issues for breast cancer patients

Often for breast cancer patients, there may be an additional component to their cognitive responses influenced by their experience of breast cancer diagnosis and treatment. Breast cancer patients might perceive their hot flushes as particularly unfair given what they have already had to endure during treatment in terms of chemotherapy and radiotherapy. Thoughts, such as, '*Why me? I've already been through so much*', and '*I don't need this as well!*' can result in feelings of frustration and anger when they experience a hot flush. Some women feel anxious as they perceive the hot flushes to be a reminder of their breast cancer, since for some women the hot flushes and menopause will have been induced by treatment. Alternatively some women view hot flushes as a reminder that their endocrine treatment, such as Tamoxifen, is helping them to stay well. So one cannot make assumptions about individual reactions and meanings – it is best to acknowledge the situation and ask women themselves. In groups of women who have breast cancer this discussion is usually very supportive and useful for the participants.

A helpful approach is to normalise their anger, empathise and then reflect back what is being said; 'It does feel unfair after what you have been through'. The aim therefore is not necessarily to directly challenge the thought but to change it to a more helpful thought promoting the message of encouraging the women to nurture themselves. This can be done by asking them to consider the disadvantages of this thought (it makes them angry and upset) and then to consider a more self-supportive response to get them through the situation by thinking about *what they would say to a friend in this situation*, e.g. *'This is tough but I can cope with this'*. Within groups, some participants who reported these cognitions were still experiencing difficulties adjusting to cancer and might require additional support from other services. This is discussed further in Chapter 6 (Session 5).

GROUP WORK ON GENERATING ALTERNATIVE AND HELPFUL THOUGHTS

Session 3, Slides 12 and 13 and Handouts 7, 8 and 9 (additional worksheets)

The group can spend some time discussing their vicious cycles with a partner using the worksheets (if they wish) and Handout 7 and writing the alternative thoughts in the 'alternative thoughts' box on Handout 8. The facilitator can circulate and help people who may be stuck while doing this and also be on the lookout for examples that can be used during feedback. Some people prefer a simpler approach to this task (using Slide 12 and Handout 7 to help them to find alternative thoughts), while others like the cognitive exercises so the additional tasks in the handouts are optional, and can be read at home.

At the end of the exercise, the facilitator can ask the group to feed back their alternative thoughts. As participants are likely to experience both types of cognitive responses in different situations, this enables them to hear alternatives that perhaps were not discussed in their group or pair and to make a note of them. The facilitator can write these on the flip chart.

This work is relatively complex, particularly when people are new to it so additional time is given to review goals for this task in the next session.

BEHAVIOURAL REACTIONS AND STRATEGIES TO MANAGE HOT FLUSHES AND PACED BREATHING LINKED IN AS A BEHAVIOURAL STRATEGY

Session 3, Slides 14, 15 and 16 (Handout 11)

Behavioural management of hot flushes is likely to take up less of the session than the cognitive aspects due to the complexity of the cognitive work. In this section, a group discussion is the best way for the group to share their methods for managing hot flushes. This can start with a brainstorming session where women are asked to contribute ideas and tips that they find helpful.

The main messages that the facilitator has to communicate for the session are:

- Reducing avoidance – highlighting the vicious cycle of avoidance and anxiety to women. This can be illustrated using 'Socratic' questioning: If you leave the situation, what is the consequence then and the next time? Are there better ways of managing the situation? How does that make you feel? Link to the cognitive work, discuss how the women can deal with symptoms that occur in social situations.
- Think of practical strategies that do not require major changes to participants' daily lives; for example, not rushing, wearing light cotton layers, using humour in social situations.
- Use paced breathing at the first sign of a flush to promote a calm response. Participants should be encouraged to consciously relax their shoulders as they take a deep breath, and then to allow the flush to flow over them. Calm acceptance of the flush is associated with feelings of control and coping. It is best to try to develop an automatic response, with attention to breathing, calm response and then attention focused outwards to a task or what she is doing in the situation. We have found that women find it easier to set aside a time to work on their thoughts, rather than to try to do this in the situation; once an alternative more helpful thought has been chosen then this can become part of the automatic response. But there are no fixed rules and different people find different strategies beneficial.

The facilitator can then summarise the strategies for the women and ask them to try out a new cognitive and/or behavioural response for the following session as homework.

RELAXATION AND PACED BREATHING

Following the introduction of paced breathing from last week, the facilitator takes the group members through a short general body relaxation instruction with more time to focus on breathing. By now, participants should have developed their relaxation skills and should find that they can enter a relaxed state more easily. Therefore, the relaxation in this session is shorter with the focus on paced breathing – the attention to breathing will start earlier in the task. This can be practised during the day while going about daily tasks and can be applied in a range of situations, such as when becoming stressed or at the start of a hot flush. Linking it with specific events, e.g. taking a break, on the hour, when travelling, can also be useful. Repeated practice may lead to an 'automatic response' of relaxation when having a hot flush, and some participants report that it actually stopped hot flushes from developing.

RELAX → SLOW BREATHING → CALMING THOUGHTS

When I felt the initial hot flush sensations in my feet, I started to practise paced breathing. The hot flush did not develop any further and the sensations in my feet subsided.

Homework

Session 3, Slide 17

- Practise brief relaxation in quiet room at a specified time each day plus using *paced breathing at the onset of hot flushes* and during stressful situations.
- Continue wellbeing/stress tasks.
- Look out for thinking around hot flushes and practise calm cognitive and behavioural responses.

- Hand out a **Hot Flush Diary** and **Sleep Diary** (handout 12, asking people to monitor their sleep during the next week in order to provide information about their sleep pattern for next session).

DEBRIEF DISCUSSION OF ANY QUESTIONS AND SUMMARISE HOMEWORK

	Mon	Tues	Wed	Thurs	Fri	Sat	Sun	*Example*
1. What time did you get up out of bed this morning?								***6.15am***
2. What time did you go to bed last night? (turned the light out)								***11.00pm***
3. How many hours between going to bed and getting up? (time in bed)								***7 hrs 15 mins***
4. How long did it take you to fall asleep (hrs)?								***30 mins***
5. How many times did you wake up during the night?								***4***
6. How many of these times were due to having a night sweat?								***3***
7. How much time were you awake during the night? (i.e. add **4** to the total time awake from when awake in **5**)								***30 mins + 1 hr 15 mins***
8. About how long did you sleep altogether (hrs)? **(3-7)** (Total sleep time)								***5 hrs 30 mins***

Figure 4.1 Sleep diary

5

Session 4: Managing night sweats and improving sleep (part one)

SUMMARY OF SESSION 4

- Feedback on the past week. Review progress so far to include triggers and stress and wellbeing goals. Review homework identifying thoughts, beliefs and behaviours in relation to hot flushes, particularly in terms of social situations and issues around control or negative consequences of a hot flush. Discuss homework and goals in pairs or smaller groups and ways of overcoming barriers. Troubleshoot any difficulties. Homework: Continue to be aware of thoughts and assumptions, and to practise using a more helpful calming thought at the onset and during a hot flush, as well as behavioural responses. (30 mins)
- Group relaxation exercise. Paced breathing/role-play having a hot flush and apply calming thoughts and breathing techniques, plus using calm breathing at onset of hot flushes and before going to sleep. (15 mins)
- Managing sleep and night sweats. Review and discuss the sleep diaries (last week's homework). Provide information about night sweats and sleep and behavioural interventions including sleep hygiene and sleep scheduling. Set individualised homework related to specific goals. (Handouts 13 and 14) (40 mins)
- Debrief discussion of any questions and summarise homework (stress reducing goals, relaxation at the onset of a flush with calming thoughts, begin to work towards sleep goals). (5 mins)

Session 4, Slide 1

The fourth session introduces the first part of the work on sleep and night sweats. Participants are quite likely to have experienced a reduction in sleep quality following the onset of hot flushes and night sweats, with episodes of waking during the night. Poor sleep is often reported to be worse than the night sweats, particularly in relation to high levels of fatigue the following day.

The sleep work is informed by cognitive behaviour therapy for insomnia (Harvey 2002; Espie 2006) to provide education about sleep in terms of what is 'normal' (quantity and quality), as well as cognitive behavioural strategies. The main part of this session is based on behavioural strategies that have been found to be effective for people experiencing sleep problems. The combination of education about sleep and behavioural strategies suggested may help to reduce anxiety about sleep disruption.

What will you need?

Flip chart and pens
Handouts 13 and 14
Hot flush weekly diaries
A watch/clock

Agenda

As with previous sessions, the facilitator should display the agenda at the beginning and add any other queries or questions at the end.

Session 4 example agenda

Review Homework:
Wellbeing/stress goals review
Thinking and behaviour in hot flushes

Sleep and night sweats part one – ***Finding out about sleep***
Improving overall sleep quality

Relaxation and paced breathing
Homework setting

REVIEWING HOMEWORK AND PROGRESS

Session 4, Slide 2

Group participants spend the first 10 minutes of this section discussing their ongoing work from the first two sessions, identifying and monitoring precipitants, and implementing wellbeing goals. The aim of this is to remind participants of this work and encourage maintenance of any changes. This can be done in pairs or if the group is quite small (6–8 women) it can be helpful to have a 'go-round' so that the group keeps up with individual women's progress.

The next 20 minutes can then be spent focusing specifically on the hot flush work with participants being encouraged to give feedback in terms of identifying and modifying cognitive behavioural responses to hot flushes. Ideally, the facilitator should go round the group and get brief feedback from each person (see example below). Any common themes or difficulties can be recorded on the flip chart and addressed once everybody has had the opportunity to speak. This will involve input from the facilitator in terms of helping to identify and address thoughts, and suggest modifications. However, the group should be encouraged to participate, provide support and help group members to continue this work.

Again the key to this exercise is empathy and reflecting back the participant's discomfort prior to trying to generate a more helpful approach. If someone is having difficulty finding helpful cognitions, or argues the case for the unhelpful cognition, the facilitator can frame the exercise in terms of developing self-support in a difficult situation by reducing the distressing emotions that accompany the hot flush. It is particularly powerful when other group members offer alternatives and therefore the facilitator should invite others to make suggestions before facilitating cognitive work themselves.

The cognitive homework might not have been carried out for various reasons. It may be too complex or participants may have difficulty identifying and modifying thoughts. This is not unexpected given the complexity of the concepts and the time given to assimilate these within groups. However, the aim is to enhance understanding of the nature of anxious or unhelpful thinking (rather than give participants advanced CBT skills) which the vast majority of participants achieve. Alternatively, participants may just find the paced breathing adequate to manage the hot flush. It is worth checking this directly with participants, as often the paced breathing is adequate in helping some women to manage their flushes (see example below). If someone does want to develop cognitive skills and needs more time, the facilitator can encourage other group members to help them to identify cognitions and suggest alternatives. Homework for the group is to continue with the cognitive and behavioural work.

Example of homework feedback in session 4

Shirley had been using paced breathing at the onset of a flush but was finding hot flushes particularly problematic during meetings at work, as she often went blank in the middle of sentences as the hot flush started. This resulted in her feeling panicky due to her perception about what others would think, and she would become flustered and less able to recall what she was saying. Between Sessions 3 and 4, she had a hot flush in a meeting and forgot what she was saying in the middle of a sentence. Remembering work on social cognitions and resulting anxieties, in addition to the positive responses in the survey, she took a deep breath and asked her colleagues to come back to her in a minute. Her colleagues were fine about this and did not ask any questions. This gave her time to gather her thoughts and continue with what she had been talking about later in the meeting. Shirley felt that this had gone well and was now considerably less anxious about the prospect of having a hot flush during meetings.

GROUP PACED BREATHING EXERCISE – PACED BREATHING/ ROLE-PLAY HAVING A HOT FLUSH

This week the group practise relaxation and specifically paced breathing. By now, group members should be well practised with relaxation and paced breathing and the vast majority will be able to implement this in circumstances that are not particularly relaxing. The idea of this exercise is to encourage them to practise paced breathing at the onset of a flush. Before beginning the exercise, the group can give feedback about the relaxation and paced breathing, providing an opportunity for the group and facilitator to troubleshoot any difficulties.

The facilitator can dim the lights and ask participants to close their eyes while they talk through a paced breathing role-play. This can involve:

'Sitting in the chair, notice how your body feels. Gently go through the parts of the body from your feet, legs, stomach, chest to your shoulders, arms, neck and head . . . notice any tension then breathe into that part of the body and let yourself relax. Wait a few minutes. Then focus on calm breathing for 5–10 breaths . . . then gradually imagine a hot flush rising – noticing the flush – and then let your shoulders relax and breathe through the flush and let it flow over you. End the practice by breathing and relaxing the whole body.'

At the end of the exercise, the group can discuss their experience and also their preferences for using calming thoughts at the start of the flush. Feedback about specific preferences and strategies is helpful for others. This enables the facilitator to communicate the options available to participants when implementing paced breathing at the start of a flush; either to apply calming thoughts generated following last week's session, or to focus exclusively on the breathing. The facilitator's role is to reinforce helpful strategies and encourage participants to implement the strategies that they find most useful.

RELAX → SLOW BREATHING → CALMING THOUGHTS

MANAGING SLEEP AND NIGHT SWEATS – REVIEW SLEEP DIARIES (LAST WEEK'S HOMEWORK). INFORMATION ABOUT SLEEP AND BEHAVIOURAL INTERVENTIONS INCLUDING SLEEP HYGIENE AND SLEEP SCHEDULING. SET SPECIFIC GOALS

Session 4, Slide 3 (Handouts 13 and 14)

Before beginning the psycho-education and behavioural work, the facilitator gives an overview of the interventions for night sweats and sleep as they are divided over two sessions. Some women will be keen for help with night sweats but the foundations of this are in basic sleep strategies and reducing anxiety about missed sleep. Therefore this session is an important component of managing the impact of night sweats without directly focusing on them.

Sample explanation

Disrupted sleep can be very distressing, though we can often manage on less sleep than we think. Night sweats can wake women up at night but the aim here is to help you to deal with them calmly, to get into an automatic routine if you are woken and to use the information in this section to deal with overly negative reactions. We'll start off by finding out a bit more about sleep to help us to understand individual sleep needs and the factors that impact on getting to sleep, staying asleep and how we feel the following day. This work will set the foundations for managing night sweats by providing strategies to enhance sleep quality overall and help us to manage when we haven't had as much sleep as we would like.

Sleep diaries review

Session 4, Slide 4

The aim of the sleep diaries is to enable participants to monitor their sleep and identify specific patterns of waking or sleep difficulties. They can be encouraged to reflect on what they have noticed about their sleep in the diary. This can be done in pairs with each pair feeding back, which is preferable as people get to know each other better. Alternatively, the facilitator can go around the group and get individual feedback, or ask people to share observations with the group, which can be recorded on the flip chart.

Specifically, participants should be asked to feed back if there was anything that surprised them about their diaries. Often group members notice that they are getting more sleep than they realised, or are able to identify patterns of specific times when they wake up. The other main information for the facilitator to draw out is how participants cope with sleep difficulties at night, and how they manage any tiredness the next day. The facilitator is then aware of which participants may be using less helpful strategies to cope with sleep difficulties (drinking coffee late in the evening, going to bed too early to make up for missed sleep, lying in bed and worrying). Counterproductive strategies to cope with daytime tiredness can be identified by the facilitator (cancelling daytime activities, napping, going to bed extra early the following night) as these are also covered during the session. The facilitator can then use this information to help participants identify specific strategies at the end of the session.

Session 4, Slide 5

The facilitator can then summarise the sleep diary feedback on the flip chart before introducing the topics that will be covered within the next two sessions using Slide 5. This illustrates to participants that there is a broad range of options available to them and, if the session is split over two sessions, encourages them to attend both sessions in order to get the most out of the sleep work.

Psycho-education of sleep basics

Session 4, Slide 6

The facilitator begins this section by introducing group members to the mechanics of sleep, specifically sleep cycles and the different types of sleep; rapid eye movement (REM) and non REM.

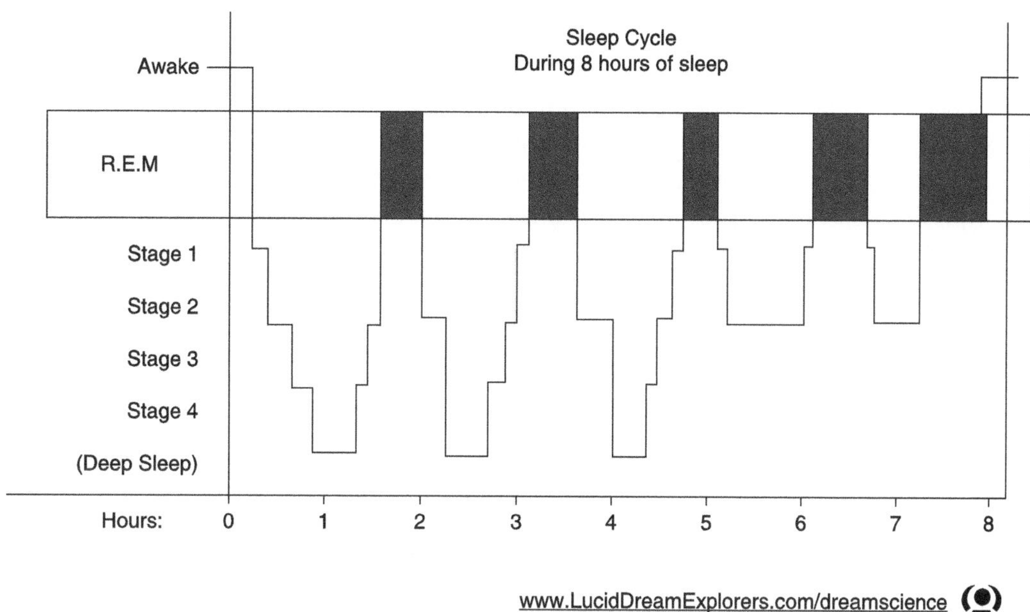

Figure 5.1 Stages of sleep (source: http://ygraph.com/chart/2076)

Talking through the diagram, and giving participants their own copy of the diagram can be helpful. A sample explanation is given below.

For the facilitator, the following important factors can help to alleviate anxieties about suboptimal sleep:

- Deep sleep occurs at the beginning of the sleep cycle and reduces as the night progresses. It is usually absent in the final third of the night. Therefore, even if the participants don't get much sleep, they will have had some deep sleep during the night, which is important for restorative processes.
- When we have missed sleep, our body automatically moves to stage 4 sleep more quickly to make up for this.
- Everybody wakes up a few times, this is normal. We may not remember waking up, whereas if you wake up and experience night sweats the period of being awake may well be longer.

The facilitator should invite participants to ask any questions, or to make any comments about the information before moving on to the slide about sleep quantity. A common query for women who have had cancer is whether sleep quality, and/or missed sleep, has a negative impact on the immune system and their health (the underlying core belief being that poor sleep might subsequently increase risk of cancer recurrence). We are not aware of any evidence of sleep influencing cancer recurrence and certainly poor sleep is not cited as a risk factor for cancer within any cancer literature (e.g. the Cancer Research UK website which has up-to-date information). This information can be cited by the facilitator, if raised as a concern.

Sleep quantity and quality

Session 4, Slide 7

The facilitator gives information that addresses the myth that everybody needs at least eight hours sleep each night and anything else is detrimental to health and performance. A study examining sleep and health data from over one million people showed that those who slept between six and eight hours per night had better health outcomes than those who consistently slept less than five and or more than nine. So while everyone differs, it seems that six to eight hours is optimal and that needing to sleep eight hours or more is a myth (Ferrie et al. 2007). This belief is very common and appears to result in a number of consequences fitting the cognitive behavioural model. Firstly, it results in feelings of anxiety if group members have anything less than eight hours of good quality uninterrupted sleep, or were having difficulty sleeping. Additionally, it also leads to a number of behaviours to compensate for missed sleep such as going to bed extra early or lying in the following day, which can contribute to the maintenance of insomnia and sleep difficulties. By addressing this belief, participants tend to report that they felt less anxious about getting X amount of hours sleep and as a result actually slept better the following week. This cognitive change can then be enhanced using the behavioural strategies described during the remainder of the session. A sample explanation of the sleep work is provided.

Sample explanation

Disturbed sleep can be distressing, although we can often manage on less sleep than we think. How much sleep we need depends on our age. This ranges from nine to ten hours for children but reduces as we get older. Most adults need six to eight hours per night but this varies as some people can get by on four hours a night. Research shows that between six and eight hours is the optimal amount and is associated with the best health outcomes. While there are other complex factors that can affect this, the important message is that six to eight hours is perfectly adequate. And anything less than this will be automatically remedied over the following nights when the body enters deeper stages of sleep much quicker than usual.

In terms of functioning, we are often able to complete our usual daily tasks on little sleep, as they are well rehearsed and automatic. When research has shown that poor sleep leads to impairments in functioning, it is often the case that people participating in the research are given highly complex tasks, a factor which is likely to impact on their performance. If they went about their usual daily tasks, any differences in functioning are likely to be negligible.

Revisiting the information about times when they may have less than six hours sleep is also helpful in terms of emphasising how the body naturally catches up the following night by going into deep sleep quicker. Additionally, while people perform less well on complex tasks after poor sleep, people can perform their usual daily tasks without any difficulties. Going about normal and rehearsed daily tasks requires less concentration, therefore performance will probably not be unduly affected. The facilitator may also wish to highlight that some days, regardless of sleep, people feel tired and weary but ignore the role of sleep within that. Therefore blaming a lack of sleep entirely on feeling this way is inaccurate and counterproductive as it focuses attention on sleep and can result in anxiety.

Session 4, Slide 8

Another aim of the sleep section is to highlight the discrepancy between subjective perceptions of sleep and objective measurement by providing participants with evidence that we are prone to make errors when estimating how well we have slept. The facilitator can feed back evidence and give examples of three different influences on sleep perception.

Because sleep is a different state of awareness, this affects our ability to make accurate judgements. Reminding the group of the sleep diagram and the different stages of sleep can help to reinforce this message. It is particularly helpful to highlight how it is normal to wake up a few times each night (this has been found when objective measures are used in the laboratory) but most people have no recollection of this. This demonstrates the inaccuracy of judgements and how sleep affects these, as most people would say they didn't wake up if asked. Participants are likely to have always woken up during the night but may only remember it now due to night sweats. The facilitator's aim is to highlight sleep as a different state of consciousness, which can reduce the accuracy of subjective judgements of sleep quality and quantity.

Recent research shows that most people:

- Underestimate how much sleep they get, and
- Overestimate how long it takes them to get to sleep.

Three main influences on our estimations of sleep are:

- ○ Sleep inertia upon waking,
- ○ Sleep onset when falling asleep, and
- ○ The role of worry.

Sleep Inertia: This is a subjective feeling of 'grogginess' upon waking which can last up to 90 minutes after we have woken up. It is also characterised by a strong urge to return to sleep. However, this tends to be the time when we are most likely to evaluate how well we have slept that night. Given that research shows that mental and physical dexterity can be significantly impaired by sleep inertia, any judgements we make are likely to be heavily influenced by it and therefore inaccurate.

Sleep Onset: This takes place during stage one of sleep and is characterised by absence of memories (amnesia). There are numerous examples of this which participants are likely to have experienced:

- When falling asleep during a film and then waking up to see the credits, it is pretty much impossible to pinpoint the exact time when sleep started – there is usually a window of about 10–20 minutes when this could have occurred.

- Laboratory experiments show that in the minutes before sleep registered as starting, people were unable to recall sounds that were presented to them. So even high-tech machines were unable to pinpoint the time, and the sleeping participants who thought they were awake could not recall the sounds.
- Another example is when people drop off to sleep and think not much time has passed (maybe a few minutes or so) but when they check the clock, an hour has passed.

In these examples, the sleeper thinks s/he has had less sleep than s/he actually had, so the tendency to underestimate sleep quantity is very common.

Worry about sleep, or any types of worry, can significantly influence perception of sleep onset so that people are more likely to make inaccurate judgements. It also leads to increased arousal and cognitive activity, which can make 10 minutes seem like 30 minutes and result in wakefulness.

It may be helpful here for the facilitator to make the connection between the cognitive behavioural model of stress and hot flushes and the cognitive behavioural model of sleep. Both menopausal symptoms and sleep are physiological phenomena, which are influenced by a range of factors. Therefore, participants can influence the cognitive and behavioural factors by making changes and thereby improve sleep quality and quantity.

Sample explanation

So while sleep difficulties can be very distressing, as is the case for hot flushes and night sweats, we can look at a range of lifestyle and behavioural factors that you can influence to improve sleep, and to help you to cope if you haven't got as much sleep as you would have liked to. Again, this uses a cognitive (thinking) and behavioural (behaviour) approach:

- *We can address behaviour at bedtime to maximise sleep onset and what to do if woken by night sweats.*
- *We can look at the role of thoughts, when we are having difficulty sleeping or if we have woken up, and their impact on how we feel.*
- *We can also look at daytime effects of not getting enough sleep and to reduce tiredness during the day.*

The strategies we will be covering are also evidence based and have been shown to improve sleep quality and quantity. We will start by looking at behavioural strategies initially with the aim of improving overall sleep quality. These can then be implemented as homework this week. Once changes have been made to enhance general sleep quality, next week we will look specifically at thinking and sleep, and also strategies for managing night sweats.

BEHAVIOURAL INTERVENTIONS TO ENHANCE GENERAL SLEEP QUALITY

Session 4, Slide 9 Handout 13

The information at the beginning of the session aims to encourage participants to implement behavioural strategies, which may run counter to their normal habits used to manage sleep. In this section group members are introduced to a range of practical behavioural strategies to improve sleep quality. The behavioural interventions are:

- Sleep habits and environment
- Stimulus control and associating bed with sleep
- Wind-down routine and relaxation
- Sleep scheduling
- Managing daytime tiredness (by maintaining and not reducing activity).

Improving basic sleep habits and environment is a good starting point that enables participants to introduce small and manageable changes to their bedroom environment and lifestyle. The facilitator can run though these quickly with participants; the following information can be provided linking with Slide 9:

Caffeine: Caffeine can delay sleep onset, reduce sleep duration and quality as well as altering the normal stages of sleep. This occurs when caffeine is drunk during the day and is not limited to a few hours before bedtime – caffeine can affect sleep up to eight hours later. The restless sleep produced by caffeine is particularly evident during the first half of sleep, which is when deep sleep occurs and when missed sleep is most likely to result in daytime tiredness.

Nicotine: This is a stimulant, so taken close to bedtime can lead to delayed sleep onset. Smokers may also go through nicotine withdrawal while they are asleep, particularly in the early part of the night, which can lead to disrupted sleep. Smokers also tend to have less deep sleep (stages 3 and 4) than non-smokers.

Alcohol: Drinking alcohol can alter sleep onset, reduce sleep duration and disrupt sleep stages. It reduces the amount of REM sleep we have, which can result in tiredness the following day. It also causes the body to release adrenaline as it tries to get rid of the alcohol; this can lead to waking and being unable to get back to sleep. So, if you drink alcohol, stop a couple of hours at least before bedtime and rehydrate.

Diet: Certain foods can increase the likelihood of dropping off to sleep; complex carbohydrates (wholegrain bread, cereals, wholemeal pasta, brown rice) lead to increase production of serotonin, which plays a significant role in falling asleep. A hot milky drink (apart from coffee/tea) can also enhance sleep onset as milk contains tryptophan, another neurotransmitter involved in sleep onset. Heavy meals prior to bedtime can reduce sleep quality as the body is working too hard to digest the food.

Exercise: Exercise in the morning or afternoon can help sleep onset and enhance sleep quality as the body naturally cools after exercise, which is conducive to sleep. Exercising too late in the evening warms the body and, as it can remain this way for up to six hours after exercise depending on intensity, it can be counterproductive to going to sleep.

Environmental factors

The optimum environment for sleep is cool, quiet, dark, comfortable and free from disruptions. The following adjustments can help to achieve this:

Limit light: The body naturally produces melatonin, a chemical involved in falling asleep, in the mid to late evening. A dark environment results in more melatonin being produced while bright lights can significantly limit melatonin production. Using blackout blinds or an eye mask can help maintain melatonin production throughout the night.

Body temperature and room temperature: The body naturally cools as it falls asleep and remains cooler during sleep. Facilitating this change in temperature by manipulating the bedroom environment, i.e. a cooler temperature, can enhance sleep onset and quality.

Limit noise: Noise, including a partner snoring, can impair sleep onset and sleep quality leading to disrupted sleep. It is therefore worth investing in earplugs, a fan or a white noise machine to help control environmental noise. Some people may find it helpful to use relaxation or peaceful sounds to listen to as they fall asleep.

Bed comfort: Ensuring that your bed is big enough, the mattress is not too hard or too soft, and the pillows are comfortable will help to increase comfort in bed and enhance sleep quality, minimising the chance of waking up due to discomfort.

Air quality: Fresh air circulating through the room can enhance sleep quality. Buying an air filter may be beneficial for people who may be allergic to dust or pollen, which can impact on breathing and therefore sleep.

Stimulus control – associating bed and sleep

Session 4, Slide 10

The facilitator may begin by asking participants to brainstorm activities that they do in the bedroom other than sleep to illustrate the wide variety of activities that participants use the bedroom for other than sleep. Stimulus control means strengthening the relationship between bed and sleep using a classical conditioning approach. It is increasingly common for people to have a television in the room, a telephone in their bedroom with people calling them late at night, or even using their laptop in bed to do work. If non-sleep inducing activities are done in the bedroom, the bedroom starts to become associated with activity and therefore is not associated with drowsiness and falling asleep. The aim of stimulus control is to limit bedroom activities to sleeping (and sex), and encouraging participants to go to bed *only* when they feel sleepy so that the association becomes stronger.

Another strategy is for participants to make sure that, if they are awake for longer than 15 minutes, that they do not remain in bed and they get up and leave the room to do something else, returning when they feel sleepy. This requires a lot of commitment and may not be consistent with work on managing night sweats which requires them to calmly get back into bed once they have cooled down and/or dried off so therefore it should be implemented at their discretion. However, participants should certainly be encouraged to use this approach when experiencing habitual morning waking. For example, if they describe waking early (e.g. 6am) but staying in bed for a few more hours and trying to fall asleep unsuccessfully, they should be encouraged to get up and out of the bedroom and start their day. While this may be difficult initially, participants frequently report an increase in sleep quality and quicker sleep onset times if they are able to maintain confining the bedroom to sleep.

Advice will differ regarding naps during the day depending on whether the group includes well women or breast cancer survivors. Usually naps should be avoided at all costs but breast cancer patients often report continuing high levels of fatigue at the end of treatment and find an afternoon nap can be beneficial and is essential sometimes to get them through the day. Therefore for these women, the advice should be avoid naps where possible, but if it is essential, try and have them before 3pm to avoid any risk of disruption to sleep cycles the following evening.

Sample explanation

In addition to some of the habits we described relating to lifestyle and sleep environment, there are also some other good sleeping habits we can apply to help the body get back into the habit of sleeping. By using the bedroom only for sleep (and sex), you can develop a strong association between bed and sleep which will help you to get into the habit of being sleepy when you go to bed. If you do work in the bedroom and it doubles as an office, or you watch TV in bed, the bed is associated with being alert, which is not conducive to falling asleep. Another difficulty is that if you have problems sleeping, you can start to associate bed with lying in bed and worrying, which then means that you don't sleep and you can get into a vicious cycle. So this approach is about making changes to influence your sleep habit and make sleep more likely when you go to bed.

Only go to bed when you feel sleepy. If you are not sleepy and it is close to bedtime, do something relaxing but away from the bedroom. Do your worrying in another room away from the bedroom in the daytime *otherwise bed and worrying can be associated, setting up a vicious cycle. In the morning, get up when you wake even if it is earlier than you would normally get up. Avoid lying in bed trying to get back to sleep if you feel alert. This may feel difficult at first but remember the sleep cycle work about how your body will naturally catch up the following night. You may find the first few nights you don't sleep as much as you like to but this is a sign of the body breaking bad habits and developing new ones. If you can maintain these changes, your body will adapt and you will feel the benefit of better sleep quality. Sleep easily gets into habit and sometimes needs retraining. It is similar to how your body adapts when you are jet lagged; the first few days or so, it is stuck in the old time zone but eventually over a week or so, it synchronises to the new time.*

Wind-down routine and relaxation

Session 4 Slide 11

Another good habit for participants to develop is a wind-down routine, which may include the relaxation that they will have been using since the start of the group sessions. Again, the underlying message is about developing better sleeping habits and routines which the body will start to respond to naturally, if they are maintained. As with stimulus control, the idea of the wind-down routine is to pair relaxing activities with the pre-bedtime period so the body and mind get into the habit of relaxing, making sleep more likely. Participants will achieve optimal results if they are able to do this at least an hour before bedtime and it may be useful to brainstorm some of the activities they engage in currently. This helps to identify activities that are not conducive to going to bed, and also participants who may already have established a good night-time routine may provide valuable suggestions for other people to try. Within our groups, it was not uncommon for people to do late night housework, or watch late night editions of the news and then feel distressed by something they had seen on there which then affected their ability to fall asleep quickly. Ideal activities include reading a book and having a warm bath (although not too hot as this may be too stimulating). The hot milky drink discussed in the previous section may form part of this routine. The relaxation and paced breathing can be included in this routine. Participants can also try these responses if they are woken by night sweats.

Sleep scheduling

Session 4, Slide 12

The basic philosophy of the sleep scheduling approach is more important than sticking rigidly to sleep restriction, which many participants may be unwilling to engage in, particularly if they experience high levels of fatigue following breast cancer. Sleep scheduling fits in neatly with stimulus control in terms of developing a robust sleeping routine and therefore good sleep habits. The idea is for participants to establish regular sleeping hours regardless of other influences or how tired they are feeling. This means going to bed at a similar time every night and getting up at the same time each morning, regardless of whether it is the weekend or if they have not slept particularly well. Linking in with the stimulus control work, participants may exacerbate poor sleep by:

- Going to bed too early the following night and subsequently lying awake for hours, becoming more anxious and less likely to sleep.
- Getting up later the following morning and subsequently disrupting their body clock so they find it more difficult to sleep the following night.

Sleep scheduling therefore aims to avoid the behaviour traps that people fall into after suffering from poor sleep which can lead to more poor sleep. It also avoids the potential vicious cycles that can develop when people try and compensate for missed sleep with lie-ins and early nights.

Sample explanation

Sleep scheduling links in well with the stimulus control strategy about confining bedroom activities to sleep to strengthen the sleep habit. These strategies can be used together or separately. The aim of sleep scheduling is to regulate your sleeping hours, which can help to improve the efficiency of your sleep. Sleep efficiency is the proportion of time that you are in bed and are asleep. If you are spending a long time in bed but not asleep, then your sleep efficiency is low and needs to improve. Sleep scheduling is therefore not about restricting sleep but sticking to regular hours, so try to avoid:

1. *Lying in really late to make up for lost time – which can have a knock-on effect the next night and reduce sleep.*
2. *Going to bed really early (e.g. at 9pm) to make up for missed sleep. The paradoxical effect being that you won't go to sleep any earlier due to your natural sleep–wake rhythms and therefore become anxious about not sleeping, making sleep less likely.*

3. *Altering the day to make up for lost sleep so that the day ends up revolving around sleep and subsequently makes sleep more difficult the following night.*

Keeping regular sleeping hours, even if they are not as long as you would like, means that when you get into bed in the evening, you are more likely to feel tired and go to sleep. Therefore your sleep quality should improve as your sleep efficiency will also improve.

Managing daytime tiredness

Session 4, Slide 13 (Handout 14)

This section of the behavioural work focuses on helping group members to establish strategies to manage daytime tiredness. This reinforces the message from the previous section about maintaining a normal routine *despite* tiredness and not letting sleep worries take over the day.

The cognitive behavioural approach to insomnia suggests that people experiencing insomnia tend to engage in a number of behaviours during the day that contribute to the maintenance of insomnia. Avoiding activities in an attempt to conserve energy can lead to inactivity, and possibly low mood, which again can increase feelings of fatigue. It can also reinforce attention biases about missing sleep leading to tension (and increased fatigue) and adding to pressure at bedtime the following night to 'catch up' on sleep. Participants may develop 'hyper vigilance' and look for signs of tiredness, which simply reinforces attention and makes them feel even more tired.

Conversely, continuing as normal has a number of benefits which participants should be made aware of:

- It provides a distraction from feeling tired and therefore reduces the tension associated with this. It also decreases the likelihood of developing cognitive biases that serve to maintain insomnia such as worrying about missed sleep.
- Pacing activities help to avoid the risk of becoming overtired, while enabling participants to achieve what they would like to during the day.
- Relaxation can be used to manage tension arising from tiredness. Physical tiredness during insomnia often arises from the tension and worry of not getting enough sleep. Relaxation can help to alleviate this and can help people to feel calm and refreshed if practised during the day.
- Activity and some exercise, such as a short brisk walk, can produce energy and alertness.

If participants remain sceptical they can test the advice out for themselves by rating tiredness and mood out of 10 on days when they limit activities and then re-rating it on days when they go about their daily activities as usual. This could be a homework task to implement for the following week.

To finish the section, participants can work in pairs to identify one or two changes to their current sleeping habits they can make using the information from this session. The sleep goals are written during the session on Handout 14. These can then be fed back to the group and will be a main section of homework for the next week.

HOMEWORK

Session 4, Slide 14

- Daily practice of brief relaxation at a specified time plus using *paced breathing at onset of hot flushes* and during stressful situations.
- Continue stress reducing and wellbeing goals.
- Continue to practise calm cognitive and behavioural responses to hot flushes.
- Implement sleep goals for next session.

6

Session 5: Managing night sweats and improving sleep (part two)

SUMMARY OF SESSION 5

- Feedback on the past week. Check on relaxation and paced breathing at times during the day, stress reducing and wellbeing goals. Discussion of homework relating to managing hot flushes. Encourage use of helpful coping strategies in the group. (20 mins)
- Group relaxation role-play. Practise relaxation in the group by role-playing dealing with a hot flush using relaxed breathing, with examples from the group. (15 mins)
- Sleep – feedback and discussion of night sweats and sleep management, summarising last session's focus on sleep habits and the behavioural strategies. Discuss thoughts and beliefs about sleep at night and in the daytime – and how to deal with cognitive arousal and worries. (Handouts 15, 16 and 17) (45 mins)
- Homework to continue with and update goals from previous week; practise using calming thoughts and breathing at the onset of a hot flush and to implement a sleep action plan to include behavioural strategies and cognitive work from this week. (5 mins)
- Review CBT model of menopausal symptoms and answer any questions. (5 mins)

Keep this summary near to hand to help with timing during the session.

Session 5, Slide 1

The fifth session continues the sleep work started in the previous session and focuses on cognitive strategies for sleep difficulties to supplement behavioural goals set as homework last week. Additionally, there is specific advice on managing night sweats, which participants may have already started to do following the previous session but it is helpful to reinforce strategies to help increase women's self-efficacy.

What will you need?

Flip chart and pens
Homework sheets 9 and 10 (from last week) and Handouts 15–17
Hot flush weekly diaries
A watch/clock

Agenda

The agenda can be written on a flip chart.

Session 5 example agenda	
Feedback on the previous week	***Reducing stress and wellbeing goals*** ***Thinking and behaviour in hot flushes***
Paced breathing practice	
Sleep and night sweats (part two) –	***Review last week's work*** ***Thinking and sleep*** ***Managing night sweats***
Homework setting	

FEEDBACK ON THE PREVIOUS WEEK

Homework review

- Check on relaxation and paced breathing at times during the day, stress reducing and wellbeing goals, modification of precipitants.
- Discussion of homework relating to managing hot flushes.
- Encourage use of helpful coping strategies in the group.
- Sleep goals are discussed in the sleep section.

Session 5, Slide 2

The first 20 minutes of the session focuses on reviewing existing hot flush goals and strategies and feeding back progress and difficulties. This will involve working in pairs and feeding back to the group with the facilitator circulating during the discussion time to help out if needed. As the second part of the sleep work forms the main part of the session, the review of the behavioural sleep homework from last week's session should remain separate from this review. The review also enables the facilitator to reinforce the importance of maintaining changes when managing hot flushes.

For some group members, by week five, some of the early work may have started to dwindle due to conflicting pressures, such as work or family demands, and the effort needed for behaviour and lifestyle change. Offering participants the opportunity to discuss barriers enables the facilitator to normalise their experience, while also encouraging them to maintain positive changes that reap benefits.

Specific issues that are likely to be pertinent at this point are:

Stress management work: Participants may have managed to implement initial strategies but have found these difficult to maintain, or their circumstances have changed, leading to the need for a new goal. The facilitator may wish to revisit the stress work as part of this discussion or encourage participants to do this as homework, pointing them towards the cognitive strategies and the problem-solving worksheet. If the facilitator does the latter, it may be useful to try and identify the stressful cognitions within the session so that other group members may offer alternative views and support as well as suggestions to resolve the situation. It can be helpful to set a new stress goal at this stage that can be reviewed in the final session, to encourage the person to modify existing stress goals that perhaps were too ambitious or to generate goals that are relevant to their current circumstances.

Cognitive therapy for hot flushes: Due to the complexity of cognitive work generally, it is likely that participants may find this aspect of the intervention difficult, so the level of explanation needs to be adjusted to the individual group member. Therefore, it can be useful to remind participants of the effects of their thinking. It is useful to involve the group in this discussion, so that they can provide empathy and support to the individual while suggesting solutions, which may involve their own personal experience in relation to the intervention.

Example

When Sue had a hot flush when she met up with friends, she would label herself as 'disgusting' (thinking) and reported that she would leave the situation (behaviour) as soon as possible to avoid others seeing the 'sweat dripping' from her (thinking). In Session 3, Sue had difficulty developing self-supportive statements rather than negative shaming statements and found that she was increasingly avoiding these situations, especially when they were meeting in busy places. This was discussed in Session 4. Other group members were able to feed back that their friends generally did not notice their symptoms, or that if they did, they had been supportive. One participant gave feedback regarding a workshop she had attended recently where she was sitting next to a woman of similar age. At the end of the workshop, one excused their appearance and disclosed her menopausal status. It transpired that neither of the women had noticed the other's hot flush symptoms despite them sitting next to each other all day. This helped to reinforce the role of self-focused attention. A few participants were also able to feed back that they felt less anxious about joking about their flushes and had received positive support from friends and family. The facilitator was also able to highlight the role of self-focused attention, as well as revisiting the survey answers to illustrate the former points about other people's views. While this discussion did not entirely alleviate Sue's anxiety, she was able to hear and consider alternative possibilities to her own experience and perspective in the situation. She reported at the end of treatment that she had found the support from other group members invaluable.

GROUP RELAXATION AND HOT FLUSH ROLE-PLAY

Session 5, Slide 3

This section begins with a brief group discussion where participants can feed back their own tips on implementing paced breathing at times during the day and at the onset of a flush. Specifically, it is useful for the facilitator to establish whether participants use calming thoughts at the onset of a hot flush in addition to the paced breathing or whether they find it helpful to switch attentional focus to their breathing only. A five minute relaxation/paced breathing exercise should then follow the discussion, giving participants a chance to try out new suggestions within the class. The facilitator talks through the breathing and role-play (see Session 4) – imagining a hot flush and breathing through it; letting the flush flow over and then at the end re-focusing attention on being in the room with others.

RELAX → SLOW BREATHING → CALMING THOUGHTS

MANAGING NIGHT SWEATS AND SLEEP (PART TWO)

(HANDOUTS 15, 16 AND 17)

The remainder of the session will focus on night sweats and sleep, beginning with a review of homework with the opportunity for participants to feed back progress and discuss any difficulties.

REVIEW SLEEP HOMEWORK

The facilitator asks for individual feedback on progress from each group member. The group can discuss any difficulties they had with the sleep goals and generate solutions to sleep problems. These can then be included in the homework for the next week. Specific topics to review with the group during this section are: Sleep habits and environment; limiting bedroom activities; using a wind-down routine and relaxation; sleep scheduling and regular sleeping hours; managing daytime tiredness.

The facilitator can reinforce positive changes made by group members and where possible include relevant sleep information to remind participants of the reasons for making any changes. For example, if they are keeping more regular (even reduced) sleeping hours and reporting increased sleep efficiency, the facilitator can reinforce the optimum sleep duration as being between six and eight hours, and the importance of maintaining a regular routine.

Examples of feedback

Gail *had noticed that she had no wind-down routine and would often start catching up with emails and housework tasks just before going to bed, which would then keep her up later. She would then get into bed and not be able to sleep. Gail had made two changes following the last session; she had implemented a wind-down routine which involved dimming the lights an hour before bed to prepare her body for sleep, as well as engaging in more relaxing activities. She also went to bed 30 minutes later and found that she fell asleep quicker as she was tired and drowsy when she went to bed.*

Lorraine *had also made two changes. She reported, 'I am not drinking coffee or tea after 2pm. It makes me a bit irritable but I am sleeping better'. Lorraine also started to practise paced breathing just before going to bed, which had also improved her sleep quality.*

SLEEP, NIGHT SWEATS AND THOUGHTS

Session 5, Slides 4, 5 and 6

This session focuses on the role of thoughts and the impact of these on emotions (e.g. anxiety) and physiological factors (e.g. fight or flight response), which can compromise our ability to fall, or go back to, sleep. To introduce the topic, participants can be asked to work in pairs to identify first of all how they think and feel if they can't fall asleep and lie awake, or when they are woken up by a night sweat and have difficulty getting back to sleep (Slide 4). Participants may report sleep specific cognitions (e.g. 'I'll feel terrible tomorrow if I don't get back to sleep'), or general worries about current life events such as family difficulties or work issues that keep them awake (Slide 5). As group members feed back these feelings, the facilitator can use the flip chart to record these and help to identify the accompanying thoughts using the following table as an example.

Situation	*Feelings*	*Thoughts*
Unable to fall asleep	Worried 75%	I'll only have had six hours sleep – I'll feel terrible all day!
Unable to get back to sleep after waking up	Frustrated 100% Anxious 80%	I'm not going to be able to function tomorrow or do my job. I'll be too tired to meet my friend after work.
General worries	Anxious 85%	Worries about work.

Once anxious or frustrated cognitive responses have been identified, the CBT model of stress from Session 2, and specifically the fight or flight response, can be revisited to remind participants of the physiological impact of anxious thoughts. The facilitator can present this information directly, or ask participants to think about what the physical consequences are of anxiety and frustration in terms of the fight or flight response and generate their own answers about the consequences of this type of thinking. This then enables the facilitator to present a rationale for the work during the session, while reminding participants of the cognitive behavioural model.

Sample explanation

These types of thoughts tend to upset us, and result in anxiety or anger, which cause us to become restless and agitated as the fight or flight response is activated. This is the opposite of being relaxed, especially at night when we feel less in control and subsequently these thoughts can keep us awake. It helps to be more relaxed to fall asleep.

Once this has been covered, the facilitator can discuss strategies to help the group to tackle anxious thinking around sleep (Slide 6). This will initially begin with sleep-related cognitions and then move on to strategies for more general worries. Following the sleep psycho-education from last week, some group members may have already made some headway in exploring unhelpful beliefs about sleep. They may report better sleep following the previous session after they realised they don't need nine hours of unbroken sleep to have slept 'well'. However, for other participants, some direct cognitive work is useful to reinforce the shift in beliefs and assumptions.

Addressing anxious sleep-related thoughts

Session 5, Slides 7 and 8

Often anxious thinking at night becomes polarised so participants report very negative expectations and worries about how they will function the next day (Slide 7). This is underpinned by the assumption that if they had slept, they would feel and perform really well all day long. The facilitator can use a continuum diagram such as Fig. 6.1 to draw out participants' expectations; how they expect they will perform compared with how they actually perform – i.e. do they perform 100 per cent all day everyday if they have had adequate sleep? Compared with their expectations of functioning at 0 per cent, do they actually sit slumped at their desk for example doing nothing at all (0 per cent), or did they manage to get some tasks done (higher rating). The facilitator can then draw these on the flip chart to provide an example of tackling anxious night-time thinking. The diagram relates to the common anxiety around being able to function at work. Other concerns often relate around appearance 'I'll look 20 years older/completely haggard' and energy levels 'I've got so much to do, I won't achieve anything'. It is particularly helpful to use a personal example from one of the participants.

Sample explanation

We often focus on the worst possible outcome (catastrophising!) and ignore any middle ground. Think about the last time you missed sleep and how you coped the following day. If the two thoughts above were 100 per cent true, then you would have been unable to think or do anything *at all and would sit near to 0 per cent! This seems unlikely. Whereas you may have felt tired at points throughout the day, or struggled occasionally with concentration, most likely you managed to do whatever tasks you needed to and felt reasonably okay. Realistically, you're more likely to be somewhere in the middle of this range, functioning 'well enough' – probably around 50 per cent.*

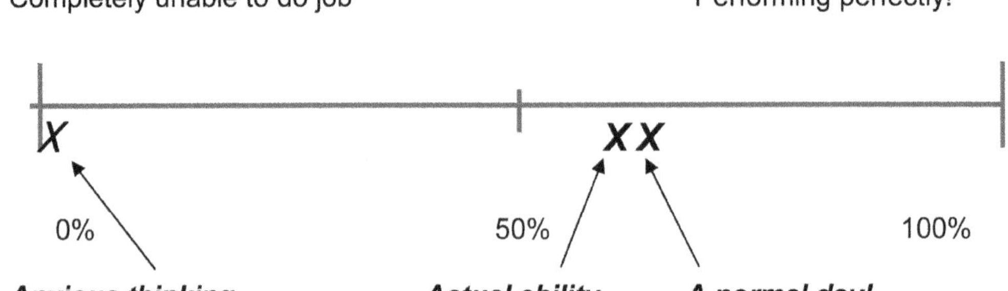

Figure 6.1 A continuum of predictions during the night about the next day compared with experience

Also even on days when sleep has been fine, we are unlikely to perform at 100 per cent all day long! So instead, try and identify a more helpful thought based on your previous experience of managing on little sleep. There are some examples:

'I can get on with usual things even if I have had a bad night's sleep.'

'Sleep problems are not dangerous or bad for me.'

'I may look a bit tired but will not have aged 10 years overnight!'

While these beliefs may be difficult to change, the group can work together to develop calmer and more self-supportive beliefs (Slide 8).

Anna *used to get very stressed about not sleeping and count the hours she would get, becoming anxious which would reduce her sleep quality. Since the sleep education group work, she started telling herself 'Whatever sleep I get will be enough' resulting in a reduction in anxiety and better sleep.*

The facilitator can help to target specific beliefs that will lead to negative automatic thoughts around sleep by reminding participants of the optimum sleep time identified within research literature, the different stages of sleep, the body's ability to catch up naturally and the influences on sleep perception and judgements. Women who have reported a change in beliefs (and subsequently sleep quality) should be encouraged to talk briefly about that to the group. Additionally, the facilitator might ask whether some of the information presented in the previous week did not support previously held beliefs.

Group members can work in pairs or small groups to address and challenge any unhelpful thoughts about sleep and generate calmer alternatives that can be recorded on the flip chart. It is important here to get participants thinking about the coping strategies they do use in this situation, as these are likely to form part of their alternative calmer thought. The facilitator may circulate during this task to help to identify participants who are having difficulty in finding alternative thoughts. The aim is to encourage group members to identify and challenge unhelpful thoughts about sleep and next day's functioning.

Dealing with worrying or stress related thoughts at night

Session 5, Slides 9 and 10

For some participants, the thoughts that keep them awake at night will be related to daytime worries or stressful personal situations. While they do not interfere with daily functioning, these worries tend to emerge at night and can compromise sleep quality. However, there are a number of strategies that are available that the facilitator can run through:

1. Practising paced breathing and relaxation – encouraging participants to focus on the breath and allow the thoughts to come and go. This will take practice and will be easier if the participant has maintained regular relaxation practice during the intervention.
2. Paced breathing can help participants to reduce their arousal levels. So as with stressful situations and hot flushes during the day, paced breathing can be used at night to help them to feel calmer.
3. Using the relaxation recording – some participants reported that they were able to go back to sleep if they listened to the relaxation CD (e.g. using headphones) when they woke in the night.
4. Using stress management strategies from Session 2 to tackle worries and stressors during waking hours (at a specific time) is a really important approach, as it helps the person to explore solutions to the problem, during the day when she will be thinking more clearly. Sleep is likely to improve once the problem has been addressed. Of course daily stresses are normal and the aim is not to be stress-free but to encourage group members to have more confidence in their own resources to manage problems that arise – and sometimes this will mean accepting or living with situations that are not ideal. The problem-solving worksheet can be used, and cognitive strategies to examine anxious thoughts within the situation and generating alternatives. This could then be their homework task for the week. Some participants may not want to share specific worries but they will still be able to talk about which strategies they can try and feed back these to the group the following week.

A useful approach is also to combine strategies: paced breathing can help women to feel calmer generally which could then be supplemented by problem-solving time during the day. The facilitator can also remind participants of the behavioural sleep work from the previous session that will help to enhance sleep quality and reduce the likelihood of getting into a vicious cycle, even if they are experiencing sleep difficulties.

Managing night sweats

Session 5, Slide 11

The final part of the session brings together all of this advice to help participants to manage night sweats. Following on from the previous week, and drawing on existing coping strategies, some group members may already have started to implement the automatic calming response. The aim is to reinforce this message and ensure that participants are aware of the cognitive and behavioural strategies which will reduce the stress of night sweats:

1. Remaining calm while cooling down, using paced breathing to maximise this.
2. Being aware of negative automatic thoughts and using strategies they have found useful previously to manage these; observing them and then bringing attention back to breathing, recognising them as anxious thinking and not fact; having calm automatic responses stemming from cognitive work during the session.
3. Returning to bed calmly and resuming paced breathing to reduce arousal.
4. Practising relaxation if this is helpful.
5. The aim is to develop an automatic routine that women can feel confident about.

Summary of sleep advice and goals

Session 5, Slides 12 and 13, Handouts 16 and 17

To finish the sleep work, participants can be asked: 'In addition to the general behavioural work from last week, which aimed to improve sleep habits, is there anything that they have learnt today or in-between sessions that they can take forward as homework this week'. This may include maintaining changes made following the last session, or it may be implementing the cognitive work from today's session to target sleep-specific cognitions or general daily worries. The facilitator can help participants develop their own sleep plans and group members can write their goals down on Handout 16.

HOMEWORK REVIEW AND ANSWER ANY QUESTIONS

Session 5, Slide 14

To finish the session and prepare for next week's session, the facilitator summarises homework for participants to carry out between this session and the final session:

- Implement a sleep action plan to include behavioural goals and cognitive strategies. The sleep psycho-education forms the rationale behind the cognitive and behavioural sleep strategies and the facilitator may emphasise this when summarising homework.
- Continue with stress reducing and wellbeing goals and precipitant modification from previous week. Maintaining changes is the main topic of Session 6 so it is crucial for participants to continue with changes from the earlier sessions.
- Continue to use paced breathing at the start of the flush and practise paced breathing/relaxation at times during the day.
- Continue to apply calming thoughts and paced breathing automatically at the onset of hot flushes and night sweats.

REVIEW CBT MODEL OF HOT FLUSHES

Session 5, Slide 15

Taking each part of the model, the facilitator can refer to the parts of the intervention that are applicable to the different parts of the model. Point out that it is the participants' perception and experience of hot flushes and night sweats in the centre of the model. The remaining boxes surrounding the central box are all the factors that influence perception and coping. A sample explanation is outlined below.

In preparation for the last session, the facilitator may want to acknowledge the large amount of information and work done over the previous five weeks and highlight how some parts may have been more useful than others. Therefore each participant will have taken different things away from each session to help them to manage hot flushes. This enables the facilitator to reinforce that the overall aim is for participants to develop self-management strategies. It also reinforces the hard work of participants who have engaged well within the groups and have made significant changes to manage their hot flushes.

Sample description

Over the last five weeks we have covered a lot of information and you have tried to implement a number of strategies and changes in a relatively short space of time. Next week we will be drawing this all together to think about how you can maintain these strategies and how they may even develop once the intervention has finished. It might be helpful now to remind ourselves of why we have been doing this work by looking at the CBT model that was presented in the first session and formed the basis of the intervention. The central box represents the factors that we are hoping to change – your perception and experience of hot flushes. This includes how many you have, how problematic they are to you, and how you cope. The surrounding boxes are all the strategies that we know can affect your experience and therefore each session has targeted one or more of these boxes with the aim of helping you to manage your hot flushes better and reduce the negative impact they may have on you.

We began in the first session by targeting the 'physiological' section of the model by finding out about the thermo-neutral zone and factors that influence this, such as stress and certain precipitants. The following session, we worked on the top box – stress and lifestyle. So you developed strategies to manage stress and enhance wellbeing, as well as starting to modify physical triggers. This work may have consequences for the physiological part of the model in terms of impacting on the thermo-neutral zone, as well as starting to influence the central part of the model. The relaxation practice also links in with these two boxes in helping you to manage stress. The third session targeted the cognitive and behavioural aspects of hot flushes to help address unhelpful thoughts and behaviours. These parts of the model were also targeted in Sessions 4 and 5 on dealing with sleep and night sweats. Developing helpful thinking and behavioural strategies has been shown in our research to impact on the middle box – your experience of hot flushes. However, as everyone is different, you are likely to have taken different things from each session. You have started the tricky part of the process by making these changes in the first place and noticing the benefits of that. The next challenge is to maintain these changes, which is the topic of the next session.

Finally next week we will have some time for general discussion, so do think if there is anything relevant to menopause etc. that you would like to discuss for next week.

Part of the final session is set aside for open discussion. This gives the group the chance to discuss topics that may not have been covered or they may want to use it as unstructured time to share experiences given the structure of the session. The group can use it how they wish. However, if there are specific topics that the group wish to discuss, the facilitator may wish to make a note of these now in case they need to prepare anything for the following week. Examples of topics chosen in our groups include: concerns relating to breast cancer patients (for groups for breast cancer patients), menopause (for women going through the menopause transition), early menopause, memory, osteoporosis, weight, sexual functioning. So it is useful to ask group members to think about any topics that we have missed and which that would like to discuss. However, time limitations only allow for a relatively brief information exchange and discussion.

7

Session 6: Review and maintaining changes

SUMMARY OF SESSION 6

- Review homework and progress overall with general discussion of what was helpful and less helpful and how to maintain changes. For example:
  - Identifying and modifying precipitants
  - Relaxation and paced breathing
  - Stress management and lifestyle changes
  - Problem-solving
  - Pacing activities and exercise
  - Hot flushes: modifying thoughts and behaviours
  - Dealing with other people
  - Night sweats and sleep: modifying thoughts and behaviours
  - Role-play: paced breathing and calm thoughts.

  Participants write down what they would like to do to maintain changes in pairs or small groups. Discuss maintaining, anticipating potential barriers, and ways of overcoming possible barriers. Group discussion of how to deal with future stresses or barriers to maintaining changes, using the CBT framework. Homework is to work on maintaining changes in the future. (Handout 18) (30 mins)
- Other menopause-related issues. The group may choose topics for part of this final session such as further discussion on one of the above topics, discussion on maintaining change in the context of breast cancer or a relevant health-related topic, such as sexual functioning, osteoporosis, weight, managing pain. (40 mins)
- Relaxation and paced breathing and calming thoughts. (10 mins)
- Goodbyes and debrief discussion. How to access help should they need to in the future. Information about post-treatment assessment and follow-up questionnaires. (10mins)

Give out diary and questionnaires and arrange follow-up assessment if appropriate to setting.

Session 6, Slide 1

The sixth session draws together the work from the previous five sessions by revisiting the CBT model of menopausal symptoms and encouraging participants to think about the changes they have made and the positive consequences of these changes. Each participant is asked to record these changes in a maintenance plan (Handout 18) for them to take away and use as a reference once the sessions have ended. The facilitator should be aware that group members might have mixed feelings about this being the last group, such as missing other participants or the regular support, and/or relief at not having further trips involving time and travel. In addition to the maintenance plan, participants are encouraged to discuss and ask questions about areas that have not been covered within the five structured sessions. The session is likely to be less formal than previous sessions with less content to cover allowing flexibility in terms of the open-ended discussion section. This session focuses on thinking about the future and ways that women can support themselves and more confidently deal with issues that might arise.

What will you need?

Flip chart and pens
Homework (Handout 16) (from last week) and Handout 18
Hot flush rating scales for each participant
A watch/clock

Agenda

The agenda can be displayed on a flip chart as always at the beginning of the session. It may be helpful to record suggestions for topics for the group discussion task at the beginning to reassure participants that they will be covered.

Session 6 example agenda

Review progress overall – what was helpful and less helpful
Maintaining changes – setting goals
Open discussion: topics?
Relaxation and breathing practice
Goodbyes

REVIEW HOMEWORK AND PROGRESS OVERALL WITH GENERAL DISCUSSION OF WHAT WAS HELPFUL AND LESS HELPFUL AND HOW TO MAINTAIN CHANGES (HANDOUT 18)

Session 6, Slides 2–4

The final homework review will focus on the work completed in Session 5 as well as opening up group discussion for anybody who is having difficulties implementing tasks between sessions. This enables other group members who may have experienced similar difficulties earlier on in the intervention to offer support and suggestions.

Important points to check are whether participants managed to modify sleep-related anxious thinking or manage worries so that they interfered less with sleep. Did they use the strategies within the session to manage night sweats, such as automatically cooling down and returning to bed using paced breathing, problem-solving daytime worries or examining unhelpful sleep beliefs? Participants may work in pairs or small groups to discuss homework and then feed back to the rest of the group so that strategies and findings are shared. The facilitator can use this opportunity to positively reinforce the implementation of helpful strategies and troubleshoot any difficulties from last week.

Once everyone has given feedback, the facilitator can ask people to feed back any difficulties with homework either from the last session or from the intervention as a whole. These can be recorded on the flip chart and have the potential to include content from any of the sessions. Common themes are ongoing difficulties in remembering to use paced breathing and relaxation, as well as daily stressors/problems that the participants may not have been able to tackle during the intervention. Once these have been recorded on the flip chart, with the facilitator's guidance the group can be asked to help participants find solutions to these issues using what they have learnt. These solutions can then be added to the maintenance plan to be tried out once the groups have finished.

Example:

Annette *identified that she was finding it difficult to do the paced breathing in a social situation. Annette told the group that she would have anxious thoughts about the flush starting and then feel silly trying to relax her shoulders and breathe deeply: 'My mind is worried because I am getting red and starting to sweat and therefore I struggle to concentrate with the breathing'. Another group member,* ***Eleanor****, offered advice on what she does in situations where it is difficult to practise deep paced breathing. Eleanor emphasised that she does not do the deeper breathing that she does during relaxation, but instead switches her attentional focus so that she continues to breathe at a normal rate but is focused on that rather than the flush. When she feels calm Eleanor then focuses back out onto the situation. This process does not take long to do and has become easier with practice.*

In our experience, when a participant has struggled to implement many of the tasks/homework in the intervention, there may be issues, such as low mood or ongoing difficulties, which can present barriers to change. The facilitator is likely to have been aware of these during the intervention and may have already taken steps to address them by, for example, referring the person to another service or encouraging them to see their GP. These issues can be more prevalent in breast cancer patients who may still be struggling to come to terms with their experience of diagnosis and treatment. It may be difficult for women to benefit fully from the intervention if adjustment issues are still very salient, whether this is distress about the diagnosis of cancer and experience of treatment, or anxiety about prognosis. Nevertheless, the intervention is likely to be helpful in relation to adjustment issues and low mood. In a recent analysis of the women who had Group CBT following breast cancer treatment, we found that those with higher levels of psychological distress before treatment actually benefited more from the treatment in terms of their hot flushes (Chilcot et al. 2014). However, if general distress and/or emotional problems persist at the end of the CBT, additional options for help can be discussed.

Example:

Beverley *felt distressed about her cancer diagnosis, the subsequent surgery and chemotherapy. In turn she experienced anger when she had hot flushes, as these were another perceived injustice arising from her breast cancer diagnosis. Typical negative automatic thoughts arising from a hot flush were, 'Not another one! This is unfair after everything I have been through, I cannot stand it any longer!'. This anger would eventually turn into low mood and helplessness that in turn prevented her from implementing homework outside of sessions. Within sessions, the facilitator and group members encouraged Beverley to draw on strengths and other strategies she was using to develop a calmer approach; e.g. 'I have been through a lot and coped with it, I am taking steps to manage my hot flushes. This one will pass soon'. Beverley valued this input but found it difficult to apply outside of sessions and was therefore encouraged to implement behavioural interventions such as relaxation and activity scheduling to help lift her mood. A significant issue for Beverley was that she was experiencing depression arising from her cancer diagnosis and needed specialist psychological support specifically to address this issue. This was discussed with her following Session 3 in a one-to-one setting where Beverley disclosed that she often felt like she was not coping but that her mood tended* *to fluctuate and she expected it to lift. The facilitator was able to discuss the emotional consequences of cancer diagnosis and treatment and explored behavioural work that Beverley could do to lift her mood. The facilitator also made a referral to the psycho-oncology service for support to address issues around adjustment.*

Complex and challenging life circumstances can present barriers to engaging fully with the self-help aspect of the intervention. There are a number of examples of this that have been encountered within our groups; such as, single parents working full-time who had children with disabilities or emotional issues, had a caring role for an elderly parent, or had additional health issues such as chronic fatigue. If not mentioned at assessment, these issues were often disclosed prior to the final session and were evident with participants reporting little change and in some cases becoming increasingly disheartened as other group members reported changes and developments. The facilitator arranged to speak to the participant outside of group time to discuss their progress and get a better idea of their life circumstances and whether additional support would be beneficial. It is therefore useful for the facilitator to have a reasonable knowledge of other services that they may be able to refer people on to. These issues highlight the importance of carrying out a thorough assessment, including general life circumstances, which can help the facilitator and the participant consider whether it is the right time to participate in the intervention.

THE MAINTENANCE PLAN

Session 6, Slides 5, 6, 7 and 8

There are several aims of the maintenance plan aside from recording what has been helpful to participants. The first is to reinforce the links between the cognitive behavioural theory to the practice of CBT for menopausal symptoms, by encouraging participants to think about what changes they have made over the previous five weeks, and why. The facilitator can make these links during the introduction and feedback of maintenance plans to the group by reinforcing cognitive and behavioural changes and by revisiting the cognitive behavioural model. Another aim of the maintenance plan is to help participants to consider circumstances that might compromise their ability to maintain changes, identify signs that this may be happening and establish an action plan to prevent setbacks. Finally, by completing the maintenance plan within the session, the participant will have a written summary that they can use in the future once the groups have been completed. The maintenance plan can be carried out with participants working on their own to complete the plan; group members then feed back at the end of this section to share useful strategies and to troubleshoot solutions should this be appropriate. A worksheet is provided for participants to complete (Handout 18).

Sample introduction

This is the last week of the programme and so we will spend some time reviewing your progress and thinking about what was helpful and less helpful to you. Everyone is different so what is important is to have a personal view about what has been helpful in terms of managing your menopausal symptoms and wellbeing over the last few weeks and how to keep this going or even take it forward. The first part of the session will therefore involve making a plan about how you might continue with the changes or goals during the next few months. We will also have a think about any difficulties you might anticipate in maintaining changes and then work

> *together to try and think of solutions to these. So what I would like you to do is put together your plan using the worksheet provided to write on (Handout 18).*

Summarising the intervention

Before completing this task the facilitator can summarise the content of the intervention (Slide 6). The list of strategies can then be left on the slide for participants to refer to while completing their plan.

- Identifying and modifying precipitants
- Relaxation and paced breathing
- Stress management and lifestyle changes
- Problem-solving
- Pacing activities and exercise
- Hot flushes: modifying thoughts and behaviours
- Social situations and control issues
- Night sweats and sleep: modifying thoughts and behaviours
- Improving sleep quality.

Participants are then asked to consider different aspects of the intervention that they have used since the beginning of the intervention. The following questions can be addressed and the facilitator can provide a rationale for these questions being included in the maintenance plan (detailed below and on Slides 7 and 8):

1. What have I learnt on my way through the course?
   What information can the participant recall that they have learnt during the intervention? What one thing has stayed with them or has been prominent to them? This could be the thermo-neutral zone, the influence of stress, the role of thoughts and behaviours on feelings, or the sleep information?
2. How have I changed the way I think, feel, or behave in response to hot flushes or night sweats?
   Leading on from the last question, participants can be encouraged to think about changes in thinking/beliefs, behaviour and feelings since starting the intervention which have been helpful in reducing the distress caused by hot flushes.
3. What might lead to a setback or be a barrier to me maintaining changes?
   Implementing aspects of the intervention tends to be easier with the regular support that group attendance provides. However, once the group has ended, participants' motivation will be an important factor in helping them to maintain any positive change or continue to develop their self-management skills. Therefore it is useful for them to consider what may get in the way of maintaining behaviours (e.g. lack of time, motivation, interruptions, family issues, feeling better, feeling tired or angry).
4. How will I know if I am having a setback?
   An important step in preventing a reduction in positive behaviour change is recognising when things have started to slip in the first place. Therefore, what signs would be early markers that indicate things are starting to slip? Participants should consider subtle signs, such as increased hot flushes, changes in thinking such as negativity or anxious thinking patterns, specific behaviours such as avoidance or withdrawal from others, as well as emotions such as stress and physical feelings such as anxiety.
5. If I do have a setback, what will I do about it?

> It is easier to plan in advance and have a ready-made action plan than to wait until they are stressed or low in mood or experiencing severe hot flushes and feel too overwhelmed to know where to start. Therefore group members are asked to consider steps they can take once they recognise the signs of a setback to get back on track. They may go 'back to basics' and implement initial changes they made during the early sessions. Reminding the group about tools from previous sessions such as stress and wellbeing and problem-solving worksheets to address new issues is also useful, as is encouraging them to refer occasionally to the materials collected over the duration of the groups.

An important point is for participants to make *realistic* plans that fit with their current circumstances and thus avoid setting themselves overly ambitious goals that would be too challenging to achieve. As well as cognitive and behavioural changes, a key aim of the intervention is reducing unrealistically high standards which in themselves tend to increase stress and lead to self-criticism. Preparing for times when things may be tough is important to help prevent feelings of failure which reduce the likelihood of getting the maintenance plan back on track. Additionally, reminding participants of the pacing/graded task approach will help make maintenance and getting back on track after a setback more manageable. It can be helpful to encourage group members to set aside a personal review session every week to think about one's own progress to maintain the rhythm of group meetings.

Once the group has discussed and recorded their plan on Handout 18, the facilitator can ask for feedback on each section of the plan. It is vital that participants write down what their plan is at this point and are able to add to it if they wish as other group members feed back their plans.

Sample explanation

If experiencing setbacks or perhaps not maintaining things as well as you have been due to other responsibilities, it is important to take a calm approach. The emphasis therefore is on not panicking or thinking you have gone back to the start and it's all been a waste of time. When approaching setbacks and maintenance of changes in a calm way, it can be useful to consider how you initially made progress in the first place. Was this by monitoring flushes or thoughts or making time for relaxation or time for yourself? Go back to basics and build up slowly over time, using the pacing approach. Break this down into small steps of what you need to do to get back on track or use the problem-solving worksheet. Think about how you coped in the past and refer to your maintenance plan. This makes resuming helpful thinking and behaviours far easier than trying to do everything at once and you are far more likely to achieve your end goal. Additionally, it is about encouraging yourself and not being self-critical.

GROUP OPEN DISCUSSION

Session 6, Slides 9–18 (as needed)

The final part of the session is open-ended and unstructured and can be used however the group wishes. It is an opportunity for them to ask questions about topics that have not been covered in the rest of the intervention, or have a more general discussion about aspects of the group intervention. All groups are different; for women who had experienced breast cancer most wanted to discuss their experiences of breast cancer treatment and coping skills informally with minimal input from the facilitator, while others had specific menopause related topics they wished to cover. In our experience, the prime difference between groups of well-women and breast cancer patients was that the former were more likely to be considering issues around psychosocial transitional aspects of menopause, and myths and consequences of menopause, while the latter will be considering issues relating to breast cancer recovery.

Specific topics, which may be useful to consider, are summarised below and on Slide 9. The facilitator should not feel that they have to be an expert in these topics although some psycho-education is provided in the slides and the following sections. S/he should emphasise that s/he cannot give medical advice but that this is an opportunity for discussion. In some groups several women might request discussion of a range of topics. The facilitator can make a judgement about how many topics to discuss and try to gain a group consensus about how to divide the remaining time as fairly as possible. The slides and information may not be needed but are included in the event that a specific topic or question arises.

Breast cancer – experience and treatments

Session 6, Slide 10

The subject of breast cancer is likely to arise in discussions since this is a key issue if shared by the group. Therefore, breast cancer survivors may benefit from considering their symptoms in the context of breast cancer and the psychological impact that diagnosis can have, especially when looking ahead. The aim of the discussion is to encourage participants to talk about their experience and share strategies for coping, which are likely to include cognitive and behavioural factors. The discussion might include normal emotions of uncertainty and anxiety during the treatment follow-up period. Additionally, this section can be used to consider adjustment following illness and how their lives may have changed (sometimes for the better as well) since their breast cancer diagnosis and treatment.

Coping with uncertainty was a topic that women who had had breast cancer often mentioned in our groups. The facilitator can normalise these emotions and offer strategies to manage the period following treatment. The main message to communicate during the discussion is that life is full of uncertainty that most of the time we avoid thinking about. While their experience of cancer and the possibility of its return is bound to raise worries about the future, behavioural reactions such as frequent checking for symptoms, hyper-vigilance, reassurance seeking, and avoidance can exacerbate anxieties and focus attention on the uncertainty, leading to negative thinking. Moreover, anxious and negative thinking patterns lead to low mood and feelings of helplessness about the future. While some of these worries may be realistic, as there is no guarantee that the cancer will not return, it is helpful for participants to develop cognitive and behavioural coping strategies to reduce emotional distress. These have all been covered in previous sessions and can help participants gain a sense of control (Slide 10).

Adjustment to breast cancer was a commonly reported issue. The facilitator may encourage the group to consider changes to their self-image since the diagnosis. Some participants may have very polarised views of themselves as either well or ill, which can lead to maladaptive strategies to 'cope' and be 'normal'. This is evident in overwork and trying to ignore the occurrence of the illness; while denial and a return to normality can be an adaptive coping response, when a group member strives to reach previous standards and levels of activity despite feeling tired and fatigued, this can be detrimental to physical wellbeing and puts them at risk of experiencing low mood. Identifying polarised thinking of healthy/normal versus ill/abnormal enables participants to consider the grey areas and the multiple factors that can contribute to their self-image.

If striving to be 'normal again' becomes exhausting, opening up discussion of a non-polarised approach can help some women to consider adaptations that may help them to manage their current physical state, as well as activities and behaviours that they can continue with regardless of their illness. The facilitator can remind them of the underlying message of self-care during this discussion and suggestions from other group members can be helpful, particularly where a participant has rigid thinking about their illness. For some, referral to a service for psychological therapy on adaptation may be beneficial.

Well-women and adjustment across the menopause transition

Session 6, Slides 11 and 12

Uncertainty is also a common emotion for women experiencing natural menopause given the biopsychosocial transition that this involves. As summarised in Chapter 1, alongside biological changes, women often experience significant psychological and social adjustments as they come to the end of childbearing years and enter a new phase of life. It can be a confusing time as media images and 'experts' tend to offer different perspectives on what women might expect to happen during the menopause, and which 'symptoms' are caused by hormone changes and which are more likely to be influenced by ageing or lifestyle. Given that many women in our groups had not discussed menopause, even with friends, they were even less likely to have discussed personal experiences, such as feelings of anxiety about a new life stage. The facilitator should therefore encourage participants to express any concerns, including anxieties or negative feelings, as well as positive feelings, they have about the menopausal transition.

Once group members have begun to share ideas and experiences, the facilitator may then encourage them to consider how they have managed other transitional points in their lives such as changing jobs, moving house, getting married or divorced, and to consider how they managed these. By highlighting the similarities between past transitions that they will all have negotiated, the group may feel more confident in their abilities to negotiate the menopausal transition despite the change and uncertainty that they feel. The message is that change can bring positive and negative reactions but that, over time, to notice the benefits and work to meet the challenge as best you can tends to be helpful.

It can be beneficial to separate the different dimensions of what happens during midlife, e.g. hot flushes, a phase of normal ageing, health problems for some, cessation of menstrual periods and the need for contraception (usually welcomed), and coincidental personal and lifestyle changes e.g. work, an ill parent, children's issues, which may or may not occur at this time.

The facilitator can help this process by asking participants to think again about the meaning of midlife and menopause. Ageing is often mentioned. Discussion of ageing and moving onto a different life stage will often reveal (overly negative) assumptions about getting older that they have not questioned such as:

'My wellbeing will decline, it's all downhill from here.'

'I will become increasingly inactive and my health will deteriorate.'

'There's no point in pursuing new interests, I'm too old!'

By highlighting the role of beliefs, the facilitator can ask participants to consider the consequences of these beliefs and to challenge overly negative attitudes to ageing and menopause. Participants can be encouraged to consider alternatives to overly negative connotations of age by thinking of people who do not fit with these beliefs, as well as other qualities of mid-aged and older women, e.g. experience, wisdom etc. This can be very relevant to women who have undergone early menopause and think that they have 'aged overnight' and are therefore 'undesirable'. Feedback from group members can help to counter such beliefs. Do they know anyone personally who has continued to develop new interests, maintain existing ones and generally thrive with age. Participants may consider people who represent different examples of ageing and may contribute towards changing attitudes towards ageing. Participants can also be encouraged to consider interests that they have not pursued or have sidelined due to other commitments such as raising a family or full-time work. This could be something they were interested in when they were younger, or have never felt they could commit time to pursuing which they may now be able to reconnect with given their changing circumstances. These discussions can also help participants to connect with and support others within the group and can lead to new decisions and changes.

Example

A very positive example in one of our groups was ***Janet*** *who talked in earlier sessions about the stressful nature of her job and the pressure to perform and be super-organised. Janet responded very well to the cognitive work and was able to identify the impact of negative thinking (catastrophising, a constant sense of urgency) on her behaviour at work and increased levels of stress, in addition to the subsequent effect this had on hot flushes. By the fourth session, Janet had put changes in place to address this pattern but had discovered that her company were restructuring and offering voluntary redundancy to all staff. She announced during the session that from the cognitive work she had identified assumptions and thoughts about having to stay at work until she reached retirement age ('I have to stay until the end', 'I have to tolerate the stress and carry on working because this is what I always thought I would do'). Janet reported that she had questioned this assumption and realised that she and her husband were in a financial situation which meant that she could consider retirement. She had decided that she did have a choice in the matter. She therefore discussed this 'revelation' with her partner and they had decided she would take the redundancy and pursue their ambition of living abroad. Janet planned to refresh her French, which is something she had always wanted to do, and they were going to move to France for a year and experience a different lifestyle.*

While this is quite an extreme example, it was helpful for Janet to feed this back to the group, as it illustrated the consequences of questioning assumptions about life stages and ageing. Janet was extremely positive about her new plans, which appeared to encourage others to reframe their views and think about the transition as an opportunity rather than a negative event. Others described looking into new hobbies now that their children had left home and many talked positively about older female role models. The aim is for the facilitator to encourage group members to be aware of the competencies and skills that they have and that they can use to deal with situations and challenges that might arise.

Example of coping with the process of transition

Rachel *had been tearful in the introductory session when asked to talk about her menopausal symptoms, as she felt overwhelmed by the menopause transition. She expressed sadness about experiencing the end of a phase in her life, as well as anxiety* *about the future, reporting that she felt 'It's all downhill from here'. Other participants within the group had agreed with her and shared her anxiety. Within the sixth session Rachel was encouraged to think about previous transitions she had managed. She talked about feeling overwhelmed by change just before she gave birth to her first child. She had worried about not working in the job she valued while on maternity leave, as well as losing her identity. However, she remembered how as soon as her child was born, she adapted and while the first few months were tough in terms of caring for a newborn baby, she had coped well and had adapted to her new circumstances. Rachel was able therefore to identify that while her current situation seemed daunting, she was looking forward to working less within the next few years and began to think about what interests she could pursue. Rachel had also recognised that she had certain assumptions about getting older that she had questioned since beginning the cognitive work leading to her feeling more confident in her ability to adapt to this new life stage.*

Sexuality and the menopause

Session 6, Slides 13 and 14

If group members wish to discuss sexual issues then the main message that the facilitator should aim to communicate is that oestrogen is one contributing factor to the issue but research has shown that the relationship, lifestyle and beliefs and expectations about sex and ageing, can have an important impact on sexual interest and functioning (Dennerstein et al. 2005).

Physical symptoms such as vaginal dryness and discomfort during intercourse can occur and are associated with lower levels of oestrogen. It may take longer for women to become aroused and there may be a reduction in sexual interest due to these changes. Vaginal dryness is associated with lower oestrogen levels and occurs more frequently during the postmenopause.

There are specific options for vaginal dryness if this is a problem:

- Vaginal lubricants can reduce discomfort with sexual activity, available without a prescription, such as K-Y Jelly, Astroglide.
- Vaginal moisturisers line the wall of the vagina and maintain vaginal moisture, such as Replens. These are used 2–3 times a week and are available at pharmacists and on prescription.
- Regular sexual stimulation promotes blood flow and secretions to the vagina.
- Taking the emphasis off intercourse for a while and exploring alternative approaches to physical intimacy can help to bring renewed enjoyment and intimacy back into sexual contact for both partners.
- Pelvic floor exercises can tone pelvic floor muscles. Instructions for these can be easily downloaded on the Internet from NHS websites or general women's health websites.
- Vaginal oestrogen cream: low-dose local oestrogen, applied directly to the vagina, can be an effective treatment, available by prescription, to relieve vaginal dryness and discomfort with sexual activity. It is best to discuss this with a doctor especially if you have a history of breast or gynaecological cancer.

Research shows that sexual interest in general tends to reduce with age, but this has been found to be associated with a range of factors such as: sexual functioning before the menopause, stress, ill health, having problematic hot flushes and night sweats, low mood, relationship status (being in a relationship or having a new partner) and partner's sexual functioning, attitudes towards sex and ageing, and cultural background (including beliefs about the importance of sex) (Avis et al. 2005). Overall, previous sexual functioning and relationship factors seem to be more important influences on women's sexual lives during the menopause than hormonal factors (Dennerstein et al. 2005). Not all menopausal women will necessarily experience this and some women even report an increase in libido and enjoyment of sex as they no longer have to worry about contraception, and also have more time with their partners after their children have left home.

Psychological factors can be addressed in a variety of ways. First, given the role that beliefs can play, the facilitator can encourage participants to consider their assumptions about menopause, ageing and sexuality. There are no fixed rules or right ways to be during the menopause in relation to sexual functioning and, of course, some women will not have partners, others will have same-sex partners and some might not be bothered by changes in sexual interest etc. For example, where are the written rules about ageing and sexuality? Are their assumptions helpful or unhelpful? An in-depth discussion is not necessarily needed; the facilitator can lead a discussion helping participants to accept differences and to decide how they wish to deal with any concerns they might have.

Highlighting the role of stress in reducing sex drive can provide motivation for women to maintain and develop stress management techniques. Behavioural approaches such as relaxation may help participants to manage anticipatory anxiety and reduce the likelihood of sex being a stressful event. Similarly steps taken to improve wellbeing, such as exercise, are likely to help people to feel better and more confident generally, and communication between partners is important so that they can address any difficulties together rather than the woman taking responsibility for sexual issues.

Body image and weight gain

Many women within the groups complained about menopausal weight gain and difficulties in controlling this or losing unwanted weight. For women who have gone through breast cancer treatment, recovery time following surgery and treatments can lead to weight increase as women tend to be less active.

Reductions in oestrogen can lead to redistribution of fat around the body, which tends to accumulate around the abdomen rather than the hips and thighs. This is due to the end of reproductive needs for fat in these areas, so while some women may remain the same weight their body shape may change which can be distressing; additionally, any weight that is gained can go straight to their stomach.

Redistribution of body fat is normal during the menopause but does not affect everyone, and weight gain is not solely due to hormonal factors. As people get older, they tend to become less active and there tends to be a reduction in daily calorific requirements, which can drop by approximately 200 calories. Therefore the solution to gaining weight or keeping further weight gain at bay is to encourage participants to eat sensibly (systematically cut out snacks or unnecessary food and see what happens) and to exercise and/or include more activity into their daily routine. Given the health implications of obesity and weight gain following menopause, which includes an increased risk of breast cancer, increased risk of heart disease and diabetes, the arguments for maintaining and increasing activity levels are clear.

This does not have to be a comprehensive exercise programme but can include activities, such as gardening or brisk walking. However, aerobic and strength training exercises are ideal as they help to replace fat with muscle, increase metabolism and are effective in controlling weight. Therefore, the group may wish to consider ways that they can introduce sensible eating and increased activity into their current routine either through formal classes or minor changes in their current lifestyle. There is evidence suggesting that weight loss, using a healthy diet and exercise, can lead to improvements in quality of life and also to improvements in hot flushes (Davis et al. 2012).

Memory

Session 6, Slide 16

Complaints of forgetfulness and poor memory are very common during midlife and participants may be particularly concerned about dementia, given its prevalence now as people are living longer, especially if a close relative such as a parent has experienced this.

Group members may be reassured to know that despite many women reporting difficulties with memory during menopause, there is very little evidence that any decline in memory is solely due to menopause. Both men and women show some age-related memory changes (and research shows that subjectively reported memory problems are more strongly associated with stress and mood than with hormone levels or stage of menopause) (Ford 2004; Mitchell and Woods 2011). This is reassuring because if people worry about not being able to remember, it can make the situation worse.

There are steps participants can take to aid their memory. It can help to be aware of situations they are prone to forgetting, or being distracted, for example, when tired, stressed or at the end of the day. Stress can have an impact on memory so anything that reduces stress, such as doing one thing at a time, should help to improve attention and memory. If you want to remember something specific linking it to a mental image can be helpful. Group members should be encouraged to not worry too much or try too hard if they can't remember something.

Osteoporosis

Session 6, Slides 17 and 18

Group members are often concerned about their risk of developing osteoporosis, something that they tend to associate with the drop in oestrogen levels at the menopause. However, osteoporosis usually only becomes a problem for people later in life due to fractures of bones. Bones become thinner with age, and the rate of change is influenced by a range of factors, such as genes, lifestyle and health. Although early menopause and being a woman are both risk factors for osteoporosis, a normal menopause does not necessarily lead to osteoporosis. Factors that also contribute to risk of osteoporosis tend to be associated with a less healthy lifestyle so this knowledge might motivate women to increase their exercise levels, which will have positive effects on wellbeing and general health.

Prevention of osteoporosis involves adequate calcium intake, regular weight-bearing exercise and reduction in smoking, alcohol and caffeine use across the lifespan, particularly among children and young women to maximise peak bone mass. Early menopause is a risk factor so it is advisable for participants to discuss hormone therapy with their doctor, if they have menopause under the age of 45. Going into menopause after this time does not raise the risk of osteoporosis. During the menopause and afterwards in order to minimise bone loss, adequate calcium is recommended together with weight-bearing exercise, such as dancing, brisk walking, jogging. A recent review of studies of exercise and bone density concluded that increasing exercise significantly improves bone density in older people (Marques et al. 2012). For further information see the National Osteoporosis Society website (www.nos.org.uk). The facilitator can advise anyone who is concerned to contact their GP for advice, for example to discuss having a bone scan or whether supplements may be beneficial.

Managing pain

Session 6, Slides 19 and 20

For breast cancer patients, aches and pains (joint and arm pains) can accompany their medication regime or continue following the end of treatment. These can have a negative impact on their mood and wellbeing. Menopausal women sometimes report joint pain as a problem as well. Therefore pain is a common choice of discussion topic. If anyone experiences persistent and troublesome pain they should be advised to seek medical help. Physiotherapy might also be advised. The cognitive behavioural approach to pain involves self-management (rather than taking away the pain) and shares similarities with approaches to hot flushes in that it acknowledges the role of thoughts, feelings and behaviours on experience of pain. Pain is stressful to live with and stress can often increase pain. This highlights the importance of stress management generally, as well as specific pain management strategies.

The facilitator can draw attention to behavioural factors that can maintain or exacerbate pain. For example, people often reduce activity in an attempt to rest the body and reduce pain. However, the consequence of doing this is that potentially enjoyable and distracting activities are reduced, and the person then focuses their attention on pain which can then lead to rumination setting up a vicious cycle (as illustrated on Slide 19). Therefore an important element of pain management involves gradually increasing activity, which may seem paradoxical but is helpful. Increasing activity and pleasurable activities, particularly if this involves physical exercise to manage stress and tension, can relieve the factors that make pain worse and provide a distraction. Overdoing activity when pain is more manageable can also lead to increased pain and a need to rest. So pacing activities, even on good days, can be a helpful way to avoid a boom and bust cycle of pain and activity (Slide 20).

Participants can be encouraged to use the cognitive work to identify overly negative or catastrophic thinking styles, which may lead to stress and anxiety and an exacerbation of pain. Participants may be asked to refer to work done in previous sessions on cognitive change to develop a calmer, self-supportive perspective and reduce the likelihood of further anxiety, which may exacerbate pain further. However, professional help should be sought if pain is persistent and/or severe.

DRAWING THE SESSION TO A CLOSE

RELAXATION PRACTICE

Session 6, Slide 21

A relaxation practice can help to draw the session to a close. The final relaxation includes 10 minutes of paced breathing with attention to breathing. The facilitator talks through a brief relaxation and paced breathing practice.

GOODBYES AND DEBRIEF

Session 6, Slide 22

The final part of this session allows the facilitator to say goodbye to group members and thank them for their valuable contribution to the groups. Acknowledging that participants' contributions are the vital ingredient for the group to work ends the sessions on a positive note. The facilitator may reinforce the need to maintain changes without placing too much pressure on the self and setting the self up for failure; participants are encouraged to continue to nurture themselves and listen to their needs, adapting their behaviour to what is taking place in their life at the time. The facilitator may also give information about contacts should participants need further help in the future and if a booster session is scheduled in, details of this can be shared here. Give out Hot Flush Rating Scale (Figure 1.3) and arrange a follow-up assessment, if needed depending on the setting.

The Hot Flush Rating Scale results can be compared with the research trial results (Ayers et al. 2012; Mann et al. 2012), in which the average Hot Flush Problem-Rating scores reduced from an average of 6/10 before the intervention to 3/10 afterwards. The facilitator may wish to schedule a booster session three or six months after the end of the group sessions but this is not essential; if practically possible it might provide motivation to maintain the changes made during the intervention.

A list of resources is included in Chapter 8 that can be referred to if women request further help or additional information or support.

Appendix: Handouts

MANAGING MENOPAUSAL SYMPTOMS

HANDOUT 1

Outline of group sessions

Each session will introduce a new topic and will build on what has been learnt during the week and in the previous session. Daily diary records are important so that we can find out how the changes you make are helping you. There will be homework and you can make individual goals for each section of the treatment.

Session 1
Introduction
Your experience of menopausal symptoms
The physiology of hot flushes
The role of thoughts, feelings and behaviour
Identifying what brings them on and makes them worse
Relaxation and paced breathing

Session 2
Identifying and modifying precipitants
Stress management and improving wellbeing
Setting individual goals
Relaxation and paced breathing

Session 3
Stress, lifestyle and problem-solving: review goals
Managing hot flushes
Examining thoughts and beliefs and behavioural reactions
Relationships and social situations
Short form of relaxation and paced breathing

Session 4
Hot flushes: thoughts, beliefs and behaviour review
Role-play dealing with hot flushes using relaxation
Managing night sweats and sleep (part one)

Session 5
Applying relaxation and changes in thoughts, feelings and behaviour to deal with hot flushes and night sweats
Managing night sweats and sleep (part two)

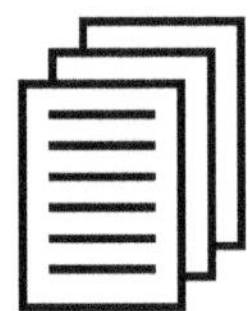

Session 6

Review
Practise managing hot flushes and discussion about maintaining changes
Sleep and night sweats
Questions and discussion
Future plans

MANAGING MENOPAUSAL SYMPTOMS

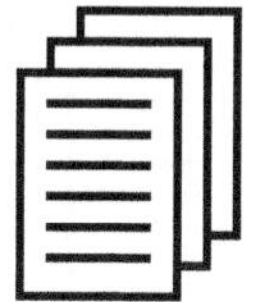

HANDOUT 2

Hot flushes, lifestyle and relaxation

Hot flushes and night sweats are the main changes experienced by women during the menopause transition – the time when menstrual periods stop. They are described as sudden sensations of heat, which spread to the upper body but they do vary a lot between women. Flushes can be accompanied by sweating and palpitations or sometimes shivering, and can cause discomfort and disrupt sleep.

Hot flushes occur when oestrogen levels are changing and adjusting to a lower level during the menopause transition. They tend to be more frequent when oestrogen reduces rapidly; for example, following surgical menopause or following treatments for breast cancer such as chemotherapy or Tamoxifen. Hormone levels affect our body temperature control mechanisms – it is as if a thermostat has a narrower range so that our bodies try to 'cool down' by having a hot flush in response to small changes in our bodies and in our surroundings. This is why reducing stress and relaxation is important. We know that hot flushes can be triggered by stimulants such as coffee, hot food and also by changes in temperature, but they are also triggered by stress. Relaxation and paced breathing can reduce general stress levels and can be used to reduce the impact of flushes when they occur.

Relaxation involves *learning a skill* – you get better at it with practice so it helps to practise every day at a regular time for 20 minutes in a quiet place. When you feel a flush coming on you can then apply the relaxation response by relaxing your shoulders and arms, focusing on your breathing and letting the flush flow over you.

It can also be useful to identify any particular lifestyle factors that trigger hot flushes for you. It could be rushing to work or drinking hot drinks or eating certain foods. Keeping a diary can enable you to identify triggers and then by making small lifestyle changes you can gain some control over your menopausal symptoms.

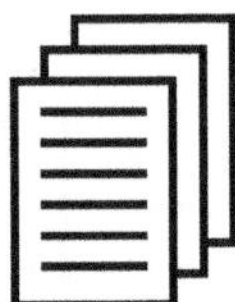

MANAGING MENOPAUSAL SYMPTOMS

HANDOUT 3

Hot flushes and night sweats: relationships between physical changes, thoughts, mood, behaviour and lifestyle

This diagram shows how HF/NS are influenced by physiological changes but also by stress and lifestyle, and by thoughts, emotions and behaviours. For example, one woman might think that people are looking at her critically when she has hot flushes and therefore avoid meeting people; she might then feel worse about herself and feel more stressed.

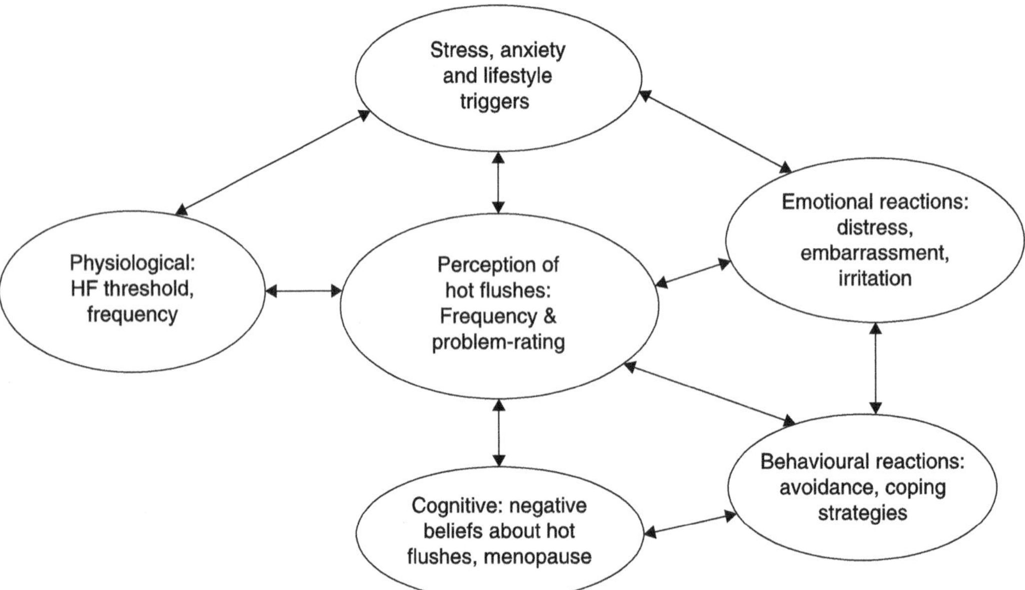

(Adapted and reproduced with permission from Hunter 2003)

MANAGING MENOPAUSAL SYMPTOMS

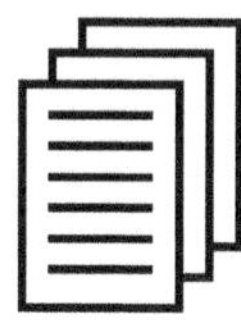

HANDOUT 4

Stress and lifestyle

Helpful strategies

- Prioritise your health and wellbeing.
- Keep a healthy balance between rest and activity by having some exercise every day if you can and by pacing activities throughout the day.
- Identify anything that is stressful or worrying and allocate a specific time to think about it and for problem-solving. It can help to write this down.
- Engage in at least one pleasant activity every day – prioritise this. It is as important, if not more so, than your other commitments.

Less helpful strategies

- Being very busy so that you are exhausted and then sleep in the daytime.
- Keeping problems to yourself and having worries at the back of your mind most of the time so that you think about them in the middle of the night.
- Not making time for yourself e.g. for exercise, relaxation or pleasant activities is unhelpful to general wellbeing.
- Avoiding people or activities.

Pacing activities and making big tasks manageable

Often when faced with a big task at work or at home, the sheer size of it leaves us *thinking* 'I don't know where to start' which can leave us *feeling* overwhelmed. As a result, our *behaviour* becomes avoidant and we tend to put things off. This stressful task therefore becomes even more stressful.

To break this pattern of avoidance, it is helpful to break the task into a series of smaller tasks and then attempt each task, one at a time with a small break in between. For example, if you have moved house and have a room full of packed boxes, instead of seeing the task as all or nothing (i.e. I must do the whole room in one go!), you can start off by unpacking one box and then having a small break. You can then do the next box and have another break.

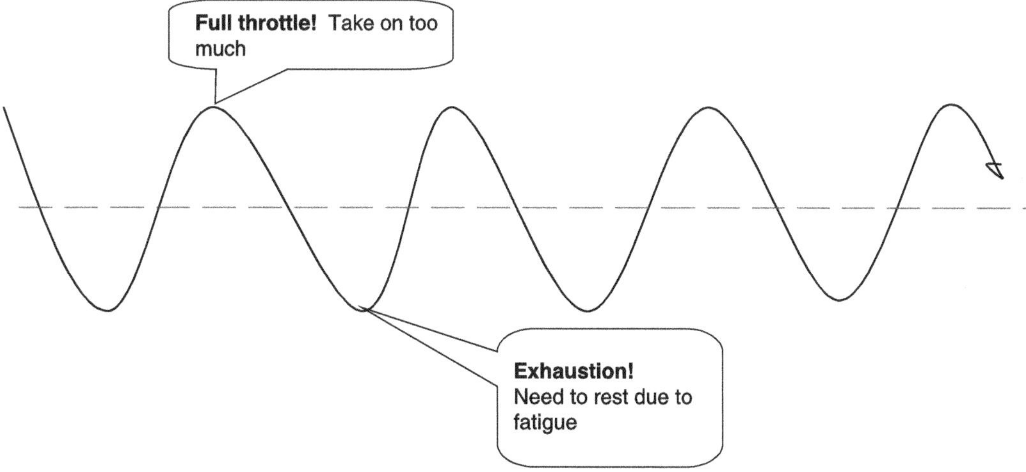

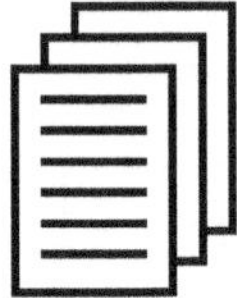

While you may not get the WHOLE task done in one day, starting to make a dent by doing little tasks helps you to *make a start*. This then reduces the *feeling* of being overwhelmed and instead you may feel pleased with your achievement. This then makes you *less likely to avoid* and more likely to carry on the next day. *Pacing* means giving yourself regular breaks generally and not wearing yourself out completely by taking too much on. It can be especially helpful if you experience fatigue as it helps people to avoid the cycle of working really hard and then having to rest as they have worn themselves out; it means doing moderate amount of activity with regular breaks, even if this is 15 minutes out in fresh air. This means that you have more stable energy levels and it helps to keep things in perspective, as it means you are less likely to wear yourself out and feel stressed.

Tackling stressful thinking

Situation that makes me stressed:

How stressed or worried do I feel out of 100?
100 = worst ever, and 0 = not at all, e.g., Anxious 75% – very stressed!

What do I worry is going to happen? Often our worries predict the worst case scenario and we believe that this is very likely to happen.

Questions to tackle anxious thinking

Is this style of thinking helping me to cope in this situation?

Yes, how does it help you to cope?

No, it is making me feel worse? Why? –

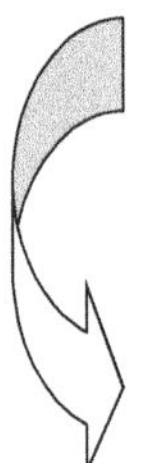

If the thoughts are not helpful, what would be a more helpful way to think about the situation? Think about a calm approach

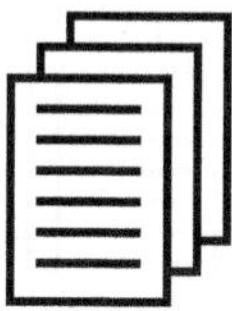

To help you think about a more helpful way to approach the situation, think about the following two questions . . .

1. Would a friend agree wholeheartedly (100 per cent) with this worried thought? If not, what may he/she advise that would help me to approach the situation calmly?

2. Conversely, if a friend had this worry, would you agree and tell her everything will go wrong and she won't be able to cope? If not, what would you suggest your friend should do or change about her thinking to help her cope with the situation?

Now, write down your calmer more helpful thoughts. Has your level of worry/anxiety reduced?

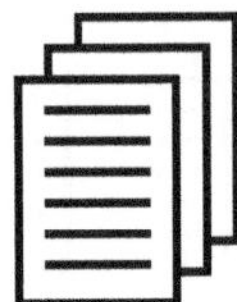

MANAGING MENOPAUSAL SYMPTOMS

HANDOUT 5

Problem-solving

We are all faced with decisions and problems to deal with on a regular basis. A useful approach is to set time aside to focus on the problem – follow the steps below:

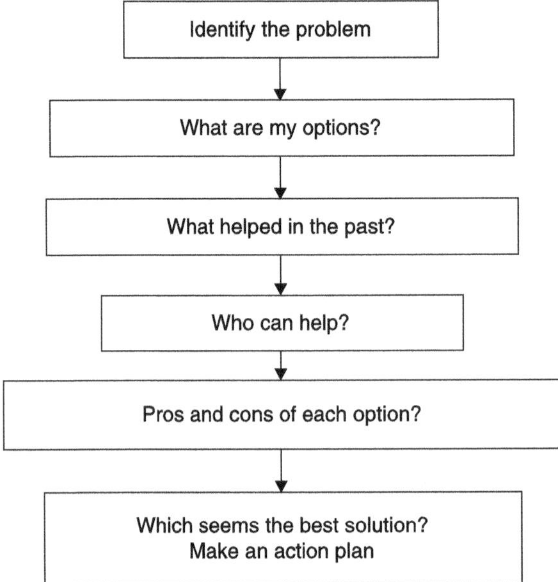

MANAGING MENOPAUSAL SYMPTOMS

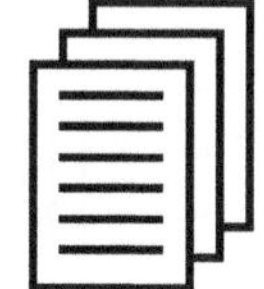

HANDOUT 6

Stress and healthy lifestyle: my goals

We would like you to think of a personal goal to reduce general levels of stress. Goals should be simple, specific and achievable. Imagine how you will put your plan into action over the next week – which means when, where and how often you will carry out your chosen behaviour.

The situation I would like to address is:

I could do this in a number of ways by addressing thinking and behaviour (write down solutions/goals in appropriate sections. You do not have to write something in every section).

Ways that I could think differently when getting stressed about this situation:

Write calmer thoughts here

My goals to enhance wellbeing are (include specific goals related to this situation and general ways to enhance wellbeing over the coming weeks):

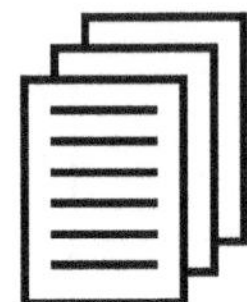

MANAGING MENOPAUSAL SYMPTOMS

HANDOUT 7

Managing hot flushes – thoughts and beliefs

UNHELPFUL THOUGHTS	MORE HELPFUL THOUGHTS
'Oh no I can't cope'	'Let's see how well I can deal with this one'
'Everyone's looking at me'	'I will notice my flushes more than other people'
'I am out of control'	'There are things I can do to control them'
'Hot flushes are bad for my health'	'There's no evidence that this is the case – most women have them'
'I'm ashamed when I have hot flushes'	'Hot flushes are part of life'
'They will go on forever'	'They will gradually reduce over time'
'I don't want people to know that I'm going through the menopause'	'Menopause is a normal part of life that I shouldn't be ashamed of'

- Check your thoughts – substitute calming thoughts instead of negative or catastrophising thoughts.
- Remember you have many different qualities as a person that are still there even though you are having a hot flush.

What would YOU think about someone else with hot flushes?

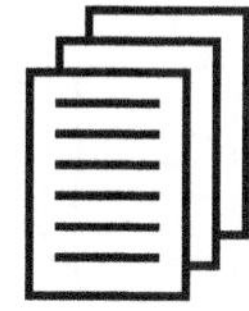

MANAGING MENOPAUSAL SYMPTOMS

HANDOUT 8

Managing hot flushes: identify your vicious cycle

Complete the vicious cycle box below.

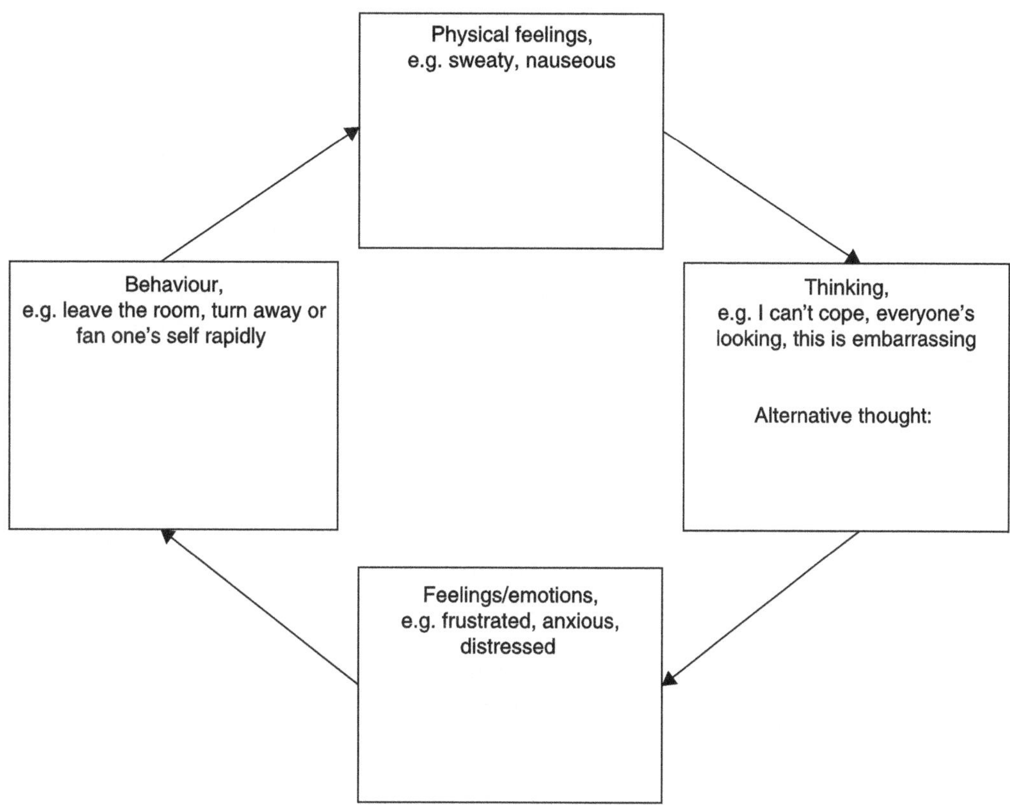

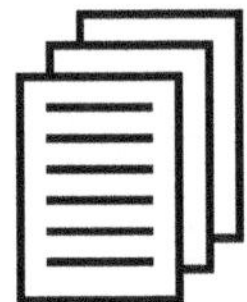

MANAGING MENOPAUSAL SYMPTOMS

HANDOUT 9

Worksheets: thinking about hot flushes

Main types of worries around hot flushes are:

- Social embarrassment (especially around men or at work)
- Lack of control.

Compared with women who reported low levels of distress around hot flushes, women with the highest levels of distress:

Have a tendency to *catastrophise* about the hot flush, e.g. 'this is out of control, I can't cope with this'; use *shaming self-labels* about their appearance (e.g. dirty, smelly, unattractive) ignoring other positive characteristics and qualities they may have; are more *self-critical* within the situation, e.g. 'I look awful, why can't I cope with these?' and report more physical sensations (indicating that their attention is focused only on the flush – which will make the sensations more powerful).

Social situations:
Embarrassment and shame arise from perceptions of what others may be thinking. Assumptions that others will be making negative judgements. These assumptions can arise from your own negative views of self and/or menopause. When you assume what others are thinking, you switch your attention from focusing outwards into the situation and instead focus it all in on yourself – this increases self-consciousness and can make the flush more intense. This also increases the tendency to judge your entire character on one aspect of the situation (i.e. the flush) rather than external factors (e.g. the other person may not have noticed or may have their own stresses that they are worrying about) or positive information about yourself.

Feeling out of control:
'Not another one!' 'I can't cope.' 'This will never end.' 'I will pass out/collapse/lose control.'

This thinking tends to be a catastrophic interpretation of symptoms – focusing on the worst outcome and on feeling unable to cope. Common thinking errors are catastrophising (these will *never* end!), 'shoulds' and 'should nots' (I *should* be able to cope), and over generalisation (I *can't* cope). This type of thinking ignores the flushes you do cope with, ignores the times when hot flushes have not interfered with your life, and makes you feel even worse, results in anger, feeling overwhelmed, frustrated or hopeless. Aim to develop higher tolerance of frustration caused by the hot flush – so, rather than saying – 'I can't cope!' 'These will never end!' – alternatives are 'I can cope using paced breathing/let's see how well I can cope with this one' as well as 'This will pass soon/my hot flushes will reduce over time.'

Can you identify any of the following in the way you are thinking about hot flushes?

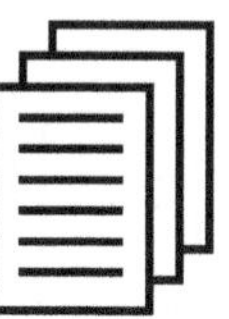

Catastrophising/fortune telling – Predicting disaster or telling yourself you can't cope (e.g. This will never end; this is taking over my life).
Shaming self-labels – Labelling yourself in a negative way (e.g. ugly, smelly, unattractive).
Self-criticism – Being harsh to yourself and talking to yourself in a way you would not talk to others (e.g. I look ridiculous).
Mind reading – Assuming what others are thinking without any evidence.
Shoulds and should-nots – Applying rigid rules to the situation (e.g. I should be able to manage this, these flushes shouldn't be happening to me).
Negative filter – Ignoring what else is going on in the situation and anything else about yourself and focusing exclusively on the flush.

Look at what you have written in the thinking box.
Does the thinking help you to cope when you have a hot flush?

Yes? How:	No, it makes me feel worse. Why?

Worries in social situations – consider if you would:

1. Negatively evaluate a friend on the same level?
2. Feel negatively towards someone who is perspiring or red in a situation?
3. Would you focus in on their flush to see how it develops and forget *everything* else that is going on in the interaction/everything you know about the person?
4. If someone did respond negatively, does that mean the thought is true or would it say something about the person who responded negatively?

Your answers to these questions should help you to think of an alternative way of thinking within the situation and highlight some thinking errors you may be making about yourself.

Worries/anger about control – things to consider when weighing up thinking:

1. Is there an alternative response other than an angry or frustrated thought/feeling?
2. Is every single hot flush like this or are you forgetting ones that you have managed well or have been milder?
3. Is there another way of responding to it that would help you feel calmer and more able to cope?
4. Are you forgetting things that do help to give you control over hot flushes (stress management, relaxation, paced breathing)?

Your answers to these questions should help you to think of an alternative way of thinking in the situation and highlight some thinking patterns about yourself.

Alternative thinking response to a hot flush:

. . . .
. . . .
. . . .

MANAGING MENOPAUSAL SYMPTOMS

HANDOUT 10

Survey results: what do other people think about hot flushes?

We conducted research to answer this question. We asked 290 men and women aged between 25 and 45 for their views and reactions to a 50-year-old woman at work with hot flush symptoms. Without mentioning menopause they were asked to identify possible causes of redness and sweating. The aim was to see if they identified the symptoms as a menopausal hot flush and whether this gave rise to negative reactions. The answers are quite illuminating!

Reasons why the woman may have a red face:

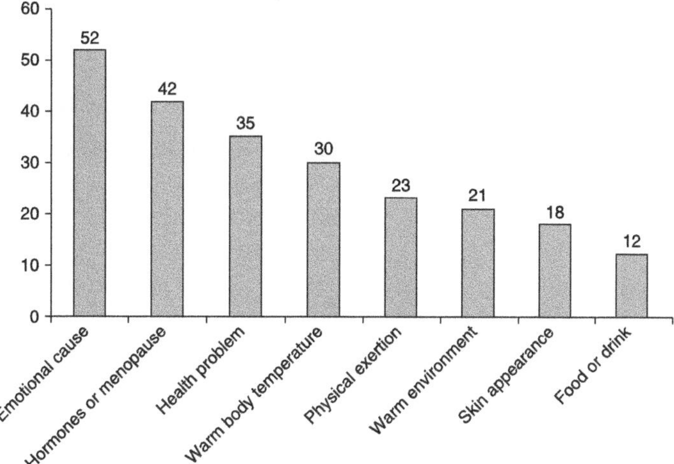

As you can see, over half thought that the woman's face may be red due to an emotional cause such as feeling stressed or a bit embarrassed. A hormonal cause or menopause was mentioned by 40 per cent with the majority simply suggesting it was due to 'hormones' or 'hot flush'. One-third mentioned a health problem such as coming down with a cold. As you can see, people gave a wide variety of reasons and did not all immediately assume menopause. These included physical exertion such as exercise or running up the stairs as the lift had broken, the room being hot, or the woman herself being a bit too hot.

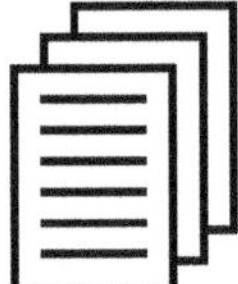

Why might she be sweating?

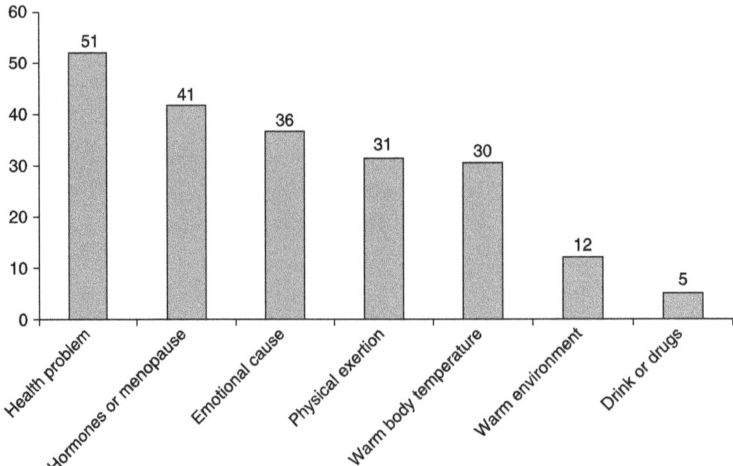

A health problem such as coming down with a cold was suggested by half of the sample. Again menopause or hormones was mentioned by just over 40 per cent with women significantly more likely to consider this a possible cause – only 20 per cent of men linked sweating to hot flushes. An emotional cause such as being stressed or embarrassed was mentioned by 36 per cent. Again people gave a wide variety of reasons including exercise and a warm room, or simply feeling a bit hot.

How would you feel towards the woman?

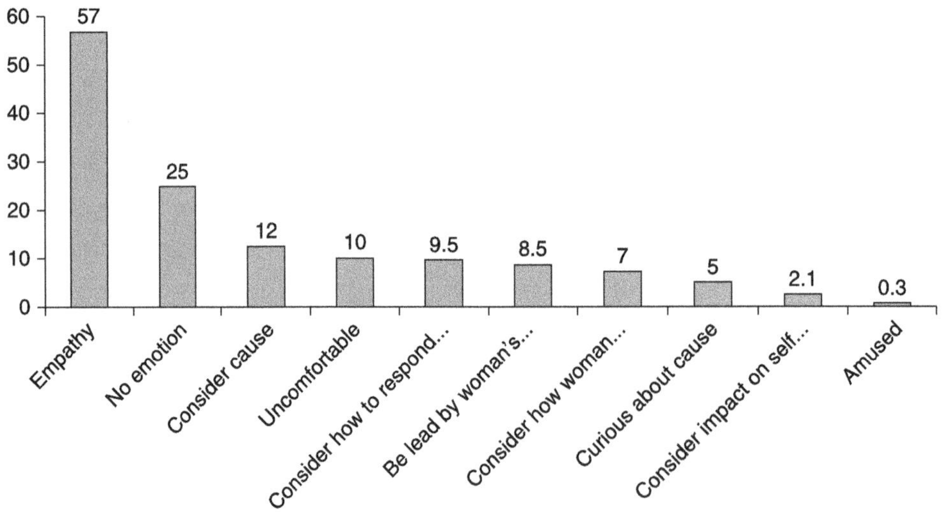

This question was asked to see if people did have negative responses that menopausal women often assume they do. Almost 60 per cent felt empathy towards the woman with 25 per cent feeling neutral. Importantly there were not any negative reactions towards the woman and often people were considering how the woman may be feeling and how to respond helpfully.

(Adapted and reproduced with kind permission of Smith et al. 2011.)

MANAGING MENOPAUSAL SYMPTOMS

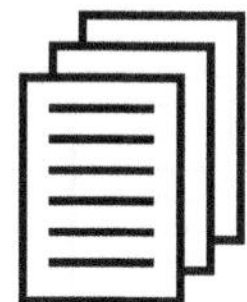

HANDOUT 11

Managing hot flushes – behavioural reactions

- Use relaxation and breathing to reduce stress on a regular basis, continue stress-reducing goals and pace activities to avoid rushing.
- At the onset of a flush let your shoulders relax, breathe slowly from your stomach and concentrate on your breathing – let the flush flow over you as you relax.
- Shift the focus of the attention to your breathing to calm yourself and then outwards to what is going on in the situation.
- Cool down with sips of water, wearing layers, carrying a fan but *try not to* rush out of social situations or avoid situations or doing things that you would usually enjoy.
- Make a light-hearted comment about it if you feel comfortable.
- Forward planning – wearing light layers, having something to distract you if in a public place (e.g. a book if on the train).

RELAX → SLOW BREATHING → CALMING THOUGHTS

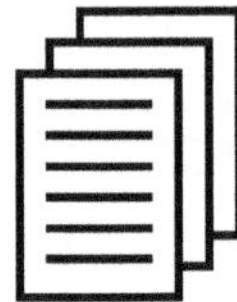

MANAGING MENOPAUSAL SYMPTOMS

HANDOUT 12

Sleep diary

	Mon	Tues	Wed	Thurs	Fri	Sat	Sun	*Example*
1. What time did you get up out of bed this morning?								***6.00am***
2. What time did you go to bed last night? (turned the light out)								***11.00pm***
3. How many hours between going to bed and getting up? (time in bed)								***7 hrs***
4. How long did it take you to fall asleep (hrs)?								***30 mins***
5. How many times did you wake up during the night?								***4 (1 hour awake)***
6. How many of these times were due to having a night sweat?								***3***
7. How much time were you awake during the night? (i.e. add **4** to the total time awake from when awake in **5**)								***30 mins + 1 hr***
8. About how long did you sleep altogether (hrs)? (**3–7**) (Total sleep time)								***5 hrs 30 mins***

MANAGING MENOPAUSAL SYMPTOMS

HANDOUT 13

Sleep hygiene principles to improve your sleep

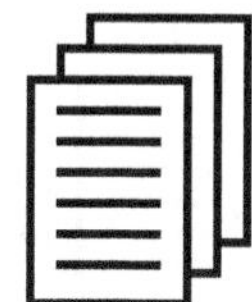

1. Helpful lifestyle and bedroom habits
   - Limit nicotine and caffeine
   - Limit alcohol
   - Manage diet
   - Manage exercise
   - Limit noise and light – keep room dark
   - Manage room temperature – keep bedroom cool
   - Improve bed comfort and air quality.
2. Sleep scheduling and stimulus control

Sleep scheduling		**Associating bed with sleep**
	AND	
Regulate the times you sleep and **stick to them**		Only use your bed for sleep and sex
		Lie down in bed only when you feel sleepy
Bed Time: e.g. 12.00 am		The idea is to keep wakefulness out of the bedroom so your body links the bedroom with sleep
Getting up: e.g. 7.00 am		Keep laptops and TVs out of the bedroom, these promote wakefulness and weaken the link between bed and sleep
Total sleep time: 7.00 hrs		Try not to nap (if you must, before 3pm, for no longer than 1 hr)
		Avoid going to bed early the following night to compensate
Sticking to these times can help you to develop a strong sleep habit.		

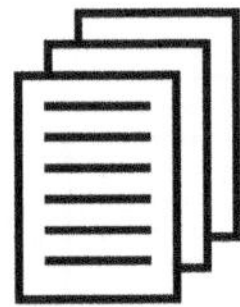

MANAGING MENOPAUSAL SYMPTOMS

HANDOUT 14

Managing sleep and night sweats

MY GOALS

We would like you to think of a couple of particular goals aimed at improving your sleep pattern. Goals should be simple, specific and achievable. Imagine how you will put your plan into action over the next week – which means when, where and how often you will carry out your chosen behaviour.

1. What?. . . . .

   When?

   Where?

   How often and how long?

2. What?. . . . .

   When?

   Where?

   How often and how long?

MANAGING MENOPAUSAL SYMPTOMS

HANDOUT 15

Managing a racing mind and breaking the cycle of worry at night

These types of thoughts can be upsetting and cause us to become restless and agitated, the opposite of feeling relaxed. It is not surprising they can keep us awake. So manage the thoughts *before* they lead to worry, don't engage with them:

- ✓ Allow thoughts to come and go, e.g. like a train passing through a station – just watch them passing by.
- ✓ Think about a pleasant, relaxing image and/or use paced breathing and relaxation.
- ✓ Think of something that will take your attention, e.g. recall the storyline from a book you have recently read, *but* nothing too detailed or complex as that will make you more alert.

If the thought does take hold this might be because the thought is associated with fears:

- ✓ Be firm in telling yourself that you will assign yourself a set 'worry time' or problem-solving time the next day (day time) to use specifically for thinking about the problem that concerns you (you can use the problem-solving approach, see Handout 5).
- ✓ Recognise the thought but let it flow over you telling yourself that you will deal with the issue in 'worry time' the next day.
- ✓ Return to relaxation, paced breathing and pleasant imagery.

Our beliefs and attitudes do affect our sleep and how we feel the next day.

What helps?

- ✓ Try not to worry about sleep – your body will make up for lost sleep in time.
- ✓ Have realistic expectations – everyone, and especially those experiencing night sweats, will have a poor night's sleep occasionally.
- ✓ Recognising that not feeling completely rested some days is normal when you wake up EVEN AFTER a good night's sleep!
- ✓ Recognise too that there are some things within your control:
    - o keeping your sleep schedule as regular as you are able
    - o cutting out negative lifestyle influences from your life and your bedroom area
    - o not napping in the daytime
    - o not spending too much time in bed.
- ✓ Get on with normal life and activities even if you have had a bad night's sleep – distracting activities can make you feel better and break sleeping habits.
- ✓ Recognise that sleep problems are not dangerous.

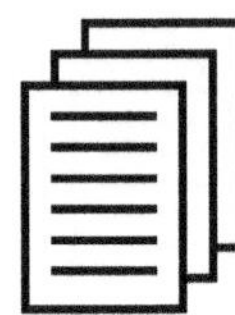

What doesn't help?

- Exaggerate the seriousness of broken sleep as this can lead to more worry e.g. 'I look 10 years older after no sleep last night' or 'I woke last night so I'll feel terrible all day'.
- Let your world revolve around sleep.
- Cancel activities as that gives you more time to worry about the upcoming night.

MANAGING MENOPAUSAL SYMPTOMS

HANDOUT 16

Managing sleep and night sweats

MY GOALS

We would like you to think of a couple of particular goals aimed at improving your sleep pattern. Goals should be simple, specific and achievable. Imagine how you will put your plan into action over the next week – which means when, where and how often you will carry out your chosen behaviour.

Ways that I could think differently when I have difficulty sleeping:

Things that I could do differently in this situation:

My goals to enhance wellbeing and sleep are (include specific goals related to this situation and general ways to enhance wellbeing over the coming weeks):

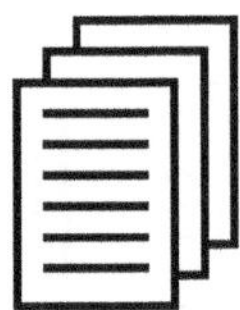

MANAGING MENOPAUSAL SYMPTOMS

HANDOUT 17

Summary of sleep advice

Behaviours

Manage environmental and lifestyle factors and maintain a regular sleep pattern:

- restrict your time in bed to your average actual sleep time,
- no napping,
- keep to the 15 min rule i.e. only lie down when tired and if lying awake for more than 15 mins you need to get out of bed until you are tired,
- keep your bed for sleep only.

Thinking

Manage worrying thoughts about any concerns you have and/or about sleep itself:

- let the thoughts flow over you (as well as the night sweats),
- don't engage with the thoughts,
- use relaxing imagery and relaxation,
- hold a flexible more accepting attitude (calming) rather than one of annoyance or exasperation (restlessness),
- arrange to problem solve during the day time for a set period of time.

Feelings

Practise relaxation to:

- reduce overall stress by providing balance to busy lives,
- as a technique to manage hot flushes/night sweats and induce sleepiness when required,
- develop a good bedtime wind-down routine.

MANAGING MENOPAUSAL SYMPTOMS

HANDOUT 18

Review of progress and maintaining changes

Review your progress in dealing with hot flushes and night sweats. Think about what was helpful and less helpful for you. Then plan how you might continue with this strategy, behaviour or goal during the next few months. For example:

- Identifying and modifying precipitants
- Relaxation and paced breathing
- Stress management and lifestyle changes
- Problem-solving
- Pacing activities and exercise
- Hot flushes: modifying thoughts and behaviour
- Dealing with other people
- Night sweats and sleep: modifying thoughts and behaviour
- Role-play: paced breathing and calm thoughts.

Write down a simple plan of the main changes that you want to maintain over the next weeks and months:

What?			
When?			
Where?			
How often?			

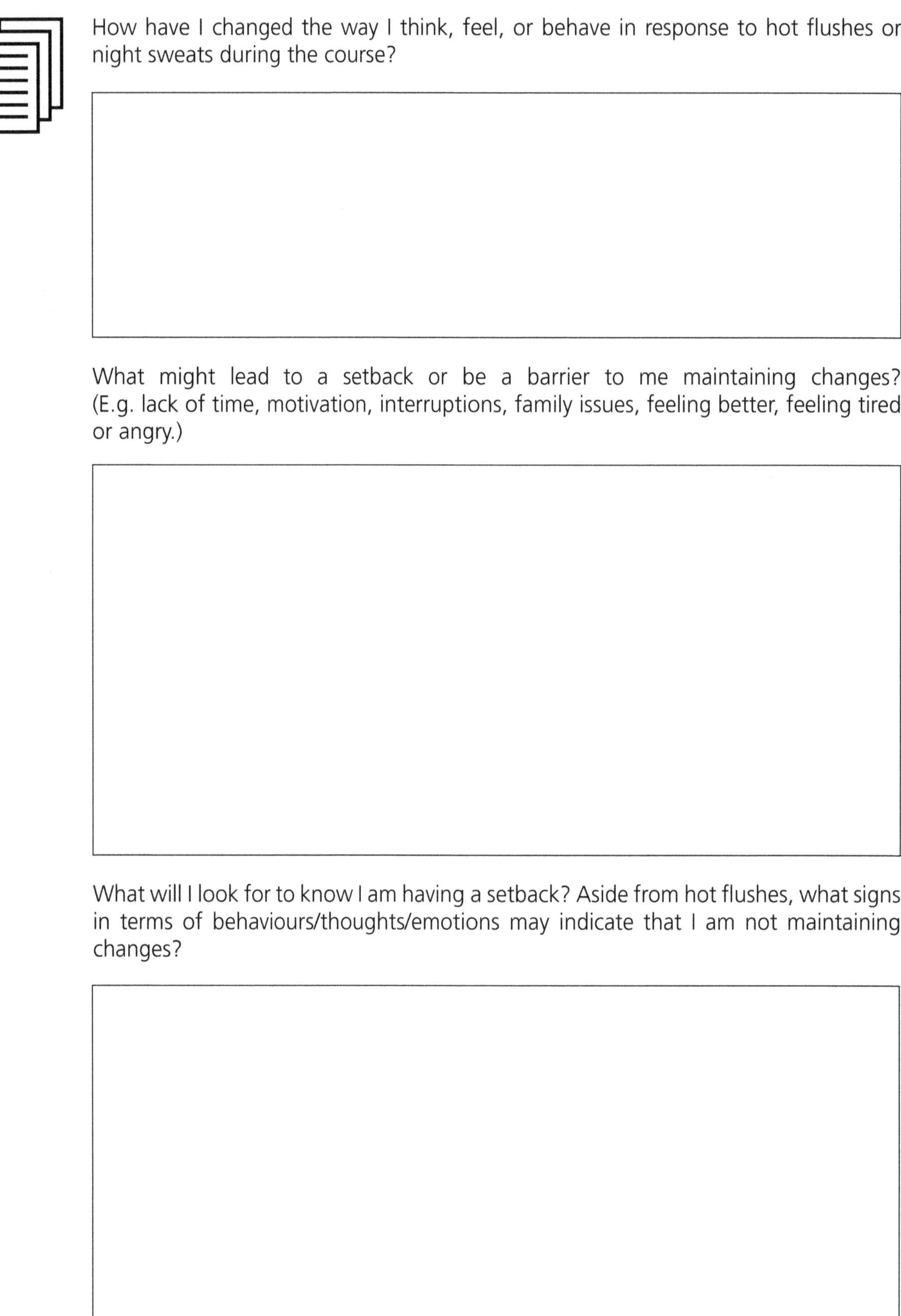

How have I changed the way I think, feel, or behave in response to hot flushes or night sweats during the course?

What might lead to a setback or be a barrier to me maintaining changes? (E.g. lack of time, motivation, interruptions, family issues, feeling better, feeling tired or angry.)

What will I look for to know I am having a setback? Aside from hot flushes, what signs in terms of behaviours/thoughts/emotions may indicate that I am not maintaining changes?

If I do have a setback, what will I do about it?

Appendix: Slides

Managing menopausal symptoms

Session 1

Professor Myra S Hunter and Dr Melanie Smith
Institute of Psychiatry, King's College London

General information and ground rules

- Groups: 4 sessions of 2 hours each or 6 sessions of 90 minutes each.
- Start and end times.
- Meet about 5–10 minutes before starting time.
- Toilets and drinks.
- Mobile phones off or on silent.
- Group confidentiality.
- Common concerns but an individual approach.
- Sharing group time and taking turns.

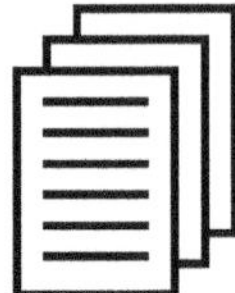

Aims of the group sessions

- To provide information and strategies to help you to deal with hot flushes and night sweats
- To use relaxation and paced breathing to reduce stress and deal with hot flushes
- To reduce hot flush triggers and their impact
- To help you to deal with night sweats and sleep problems
- To set individual goals
- To provide a supportive setting where you can learn from each other

What are your experiences of menopause?

Which symptoms are particularly problematic for you?

What are your goals for attending the group?

What would you like to address?

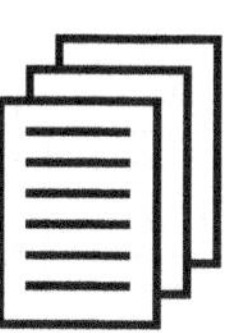

The menopause

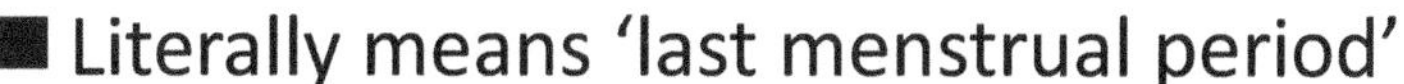

- Literally means 'last menstrual period'
- Occurs on average at age 50–51 years
- Average age of onset is 47 years
- Average duration 4 years but can last longer
- Main symptoms are hot flushes and night sweats, which affect 60–70% of women, and these can be induced by breast cancer treatments
- Symptoms experienced as 'problematic' by 20–25% of women
- Occurs at a time when there may be other life changes

Physiological mechanisms: what happens during a hot flush?

Hot flush thresholds with and without symptoms

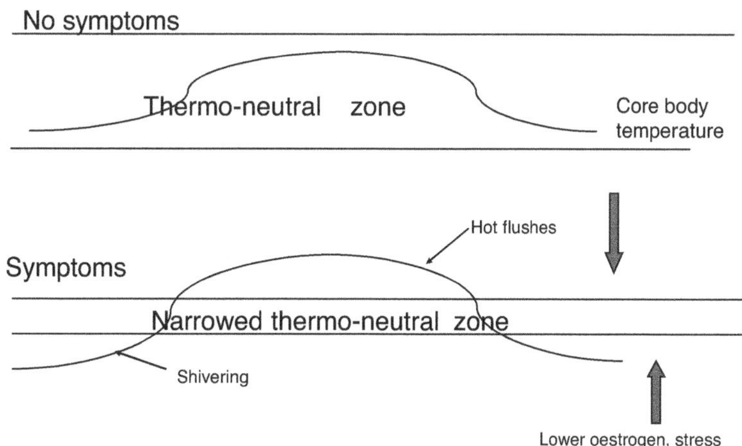

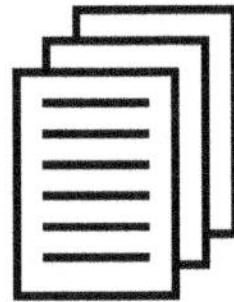

Thoughts, feelings, behaviour and physical reactions
Physical reactions
Thoughts
Behaviour
Feelings
© 2015, *Managing Hot Flushes with Group Cognitive Behaviour Therapy*,
Myra Hunter and Melanie Smith, Routledge

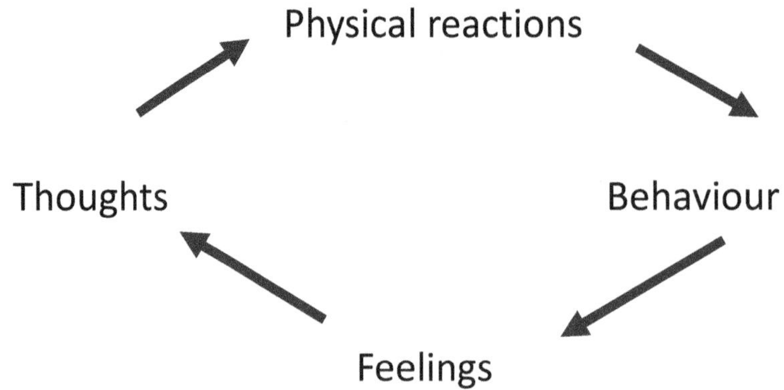

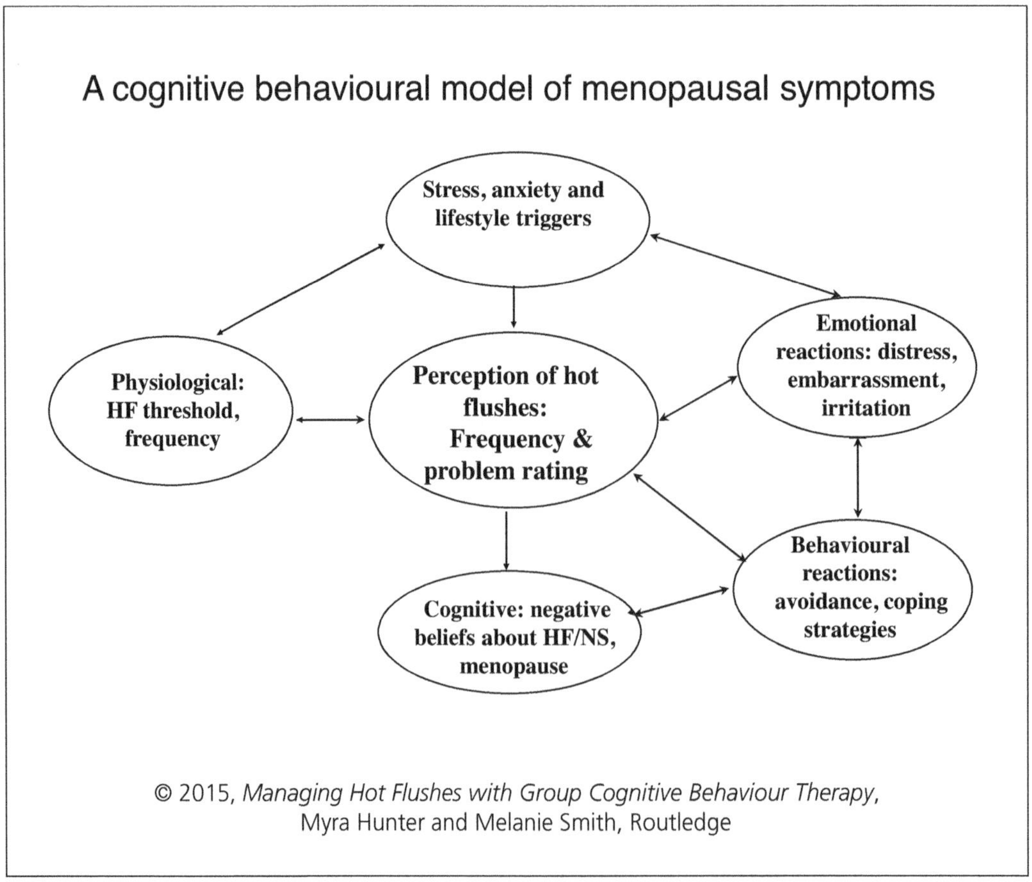

A cognitive behavioural model of menopausal symptoms
Stress, anxiety and lifestyle triggers
Physiological: HF threshold, frequency
Perception of hot flushes: Frequency & problem rating
Emotional reactions: distress, embarrassment, irritation
Behavioural reactions: avoidance, coping strategies
Cognitive: negative beliefs about HF/NS, menopause
© 2015, *Managing Hot Flushes with Group Cognitive Behaviour Therapy*,
Myra Hunter and Melanie Smith, Routledge

What helps?

- Applying breathing and relaxation at the onset of a hot flush
- Paced breathing and relaxation to widen the hot flush threshold
- Reducing stress in general
- Addressing thinking and behaviour
- Identifying and modifying hot flush triggers

Triggers of hot flushes

- Coffee
- Tea
- Hot spicy foods
- Rapid change of temperature
- Alcohol
- Rushing to work
- Hot crowded places
- Feeling angry
- Feeling tense
- Feeling overwhelmed

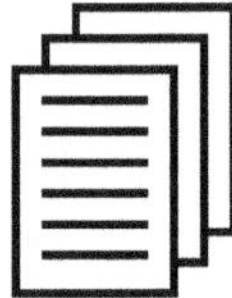

Breathing and relaxation

- Paced even breathing from stomach, called 'diaphragmatic' breathing
- Muscle relaxation: tensing and relaxing muscle groups
- Learning a skill
- Regular practice and note in diary
- Using CD and practise in group sessions

Homework

- Monitoring triggers during the week
- Begin practising relaxation every day for 15–20 mins if possible
- Note down triggers and relaxation practice in diary

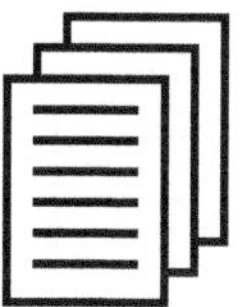

Stress management and improving wellbeing

Session 2

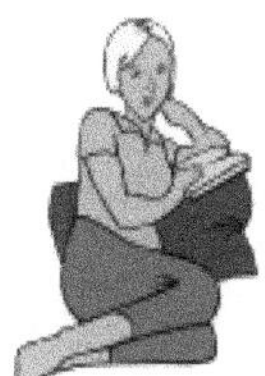

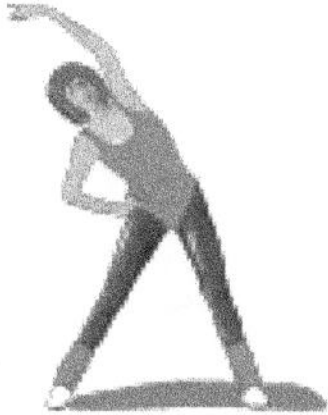

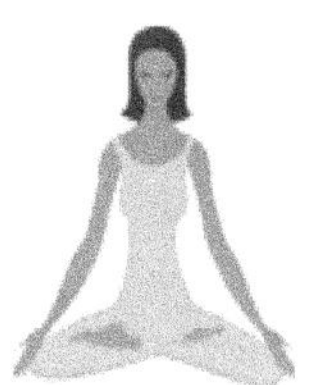

Professor Myra S Hunter and Dr Melanie Smith
Institute of Psychiatry, King's College London

Review of the week

How are you getting on with different aspects of the programme?

- Relaxation
- Monitoring and modification of your triggers
- In pairs discuss any barriers you have encountered and ways of overcoming them

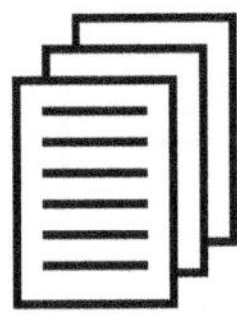

A cognitive behavioural model of menopausal hot flushes: thoughts, mood, behaviour and lifestyle

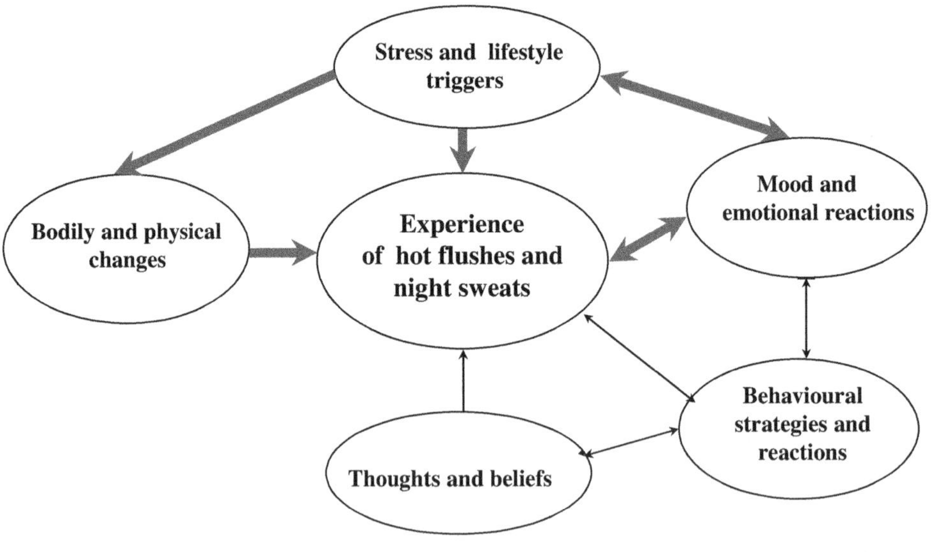

What causes stress?

- Stress is a *normal* part of everyday life
- What is stressful varies from person to person
- Stress occurs when:

A situation places huge demands on us

AND

We think that we do not have the personal resources to manage the situation

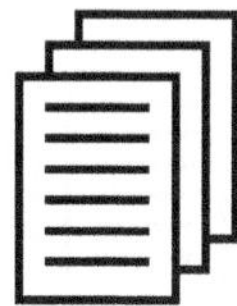

Effects of stress

- It is important to recognise the signs that you are getting really stressed
- The 'fight or flight' response

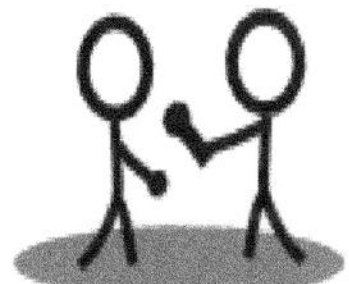

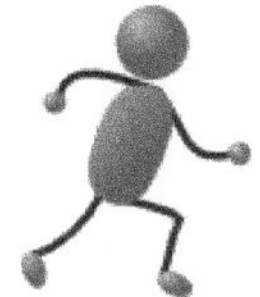

Thoughts, feelings, behaviour and physical reactions

Physical reactions → Behaviour → Feelings → Thoughts → Physical reactions

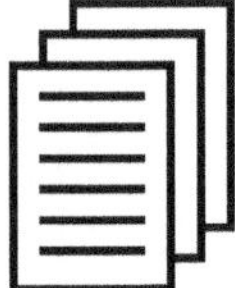

Recognising the signs of stress

- **Bodily symptoms**: tension, aches, heart racing
- **Mood**: irritability, anger, frustration, crying, venting of feelings
- **Cognitive**: Anxious thoughts, e.g. 'I'm not going to finish this!' 'I'm not good enough' 'I can't please everyone!' 'They will think badly of me!'
  - Overestimate likelihood of negative outcome
  - Underestimate ability to cope
- **Behaviour**: affects general wellbeing and the extent to which people look after themselves (working hours, smoking, drinking); withdrawing from other people and positive activities

How to reduce stress and improve wellbeing

- Prioritising own health and wellbeing
- Calmer thinking – identifying unhelpful thoughts and coming up with 'calmer' and more helpful alternatives
- Regular exercising (e.g. brisk walking, swimming)
- Engaging in pleasant activities and taking time for yourself
- Pacing activities (planning and allowing regular breaks)
- Problem-solving

Tackling stressful thinking

- Impact of anxious thoughts, e.g. catastrophic predictions on emotions:
  - Advantages of thinking this way
  - Disadvantages of thinking this way
- Consider other ways of thinking that may lead you to feel less stressed by answering the following:
  - Would a friend agree wholeheartedly with this approach to the situation?
  - What might they say to help me calm down?
  - What would you say to a friend in the same situation?

The boom and bust cycle

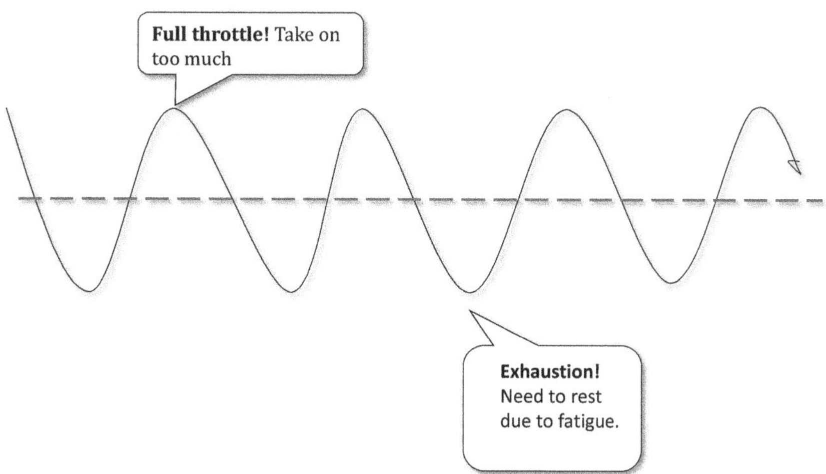

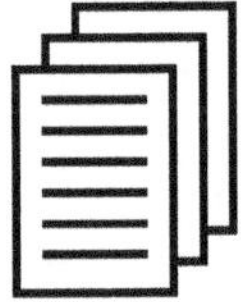

Problem-solving

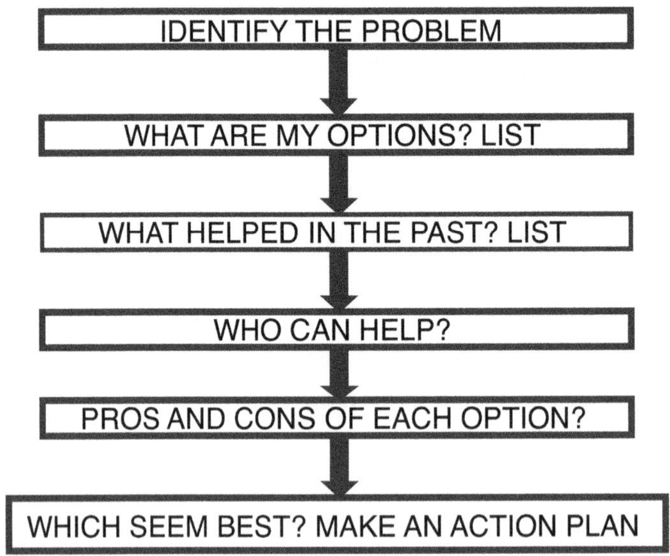

Stress and lifestyle

Helpful strategies:

- Prioritising own health and wellbeing
- Not rushing
- Keeping a balance between rest and activity (e.g. exercising every day) and pacing activities throughout the day
- Identify anything stressful and worrying and allocate a specific time for problem-solving. It can be helpful to write this down
- Identifying anxious thinking which may increase your levels of stress
- Engage in at least one pleasant activity per day

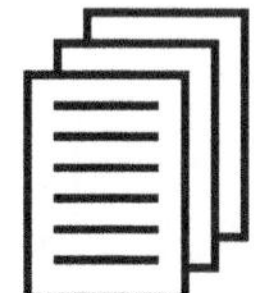

Stress and lifestyle

Less helpful strategies:

- Being very busy and exhausting yourself, and sleeping in the daytime
- Keeping problems to yourself, bottling up worries and keeping them at the back of your mind most of the time
- Not making time for yourself for exercise, relaxation or pleasant activities
- Avoiding people or activities because of menopausal symptoms

Reducing stress/effects of stress

- How could you reduce stress for yourself?
- In pairs identify and discuss own personal goals for reducing stress
- Goals should be specific and measurable:

  'going for a 15 minute walk once a day', rather than 'walking more', setting aside time to problem solve an ongoing stress, or 'identifying thinking errors and coming up with an alternative'
- Feed back your personal goals to the group

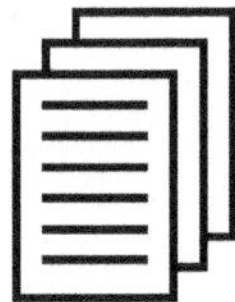

Group relaxation and homework

- Practising relaxation and focus on breathing at the onset of a flush
- Continue to practise daily
- Monitoring and modify triggers during the week
- Carry out stress/wellbeing goal

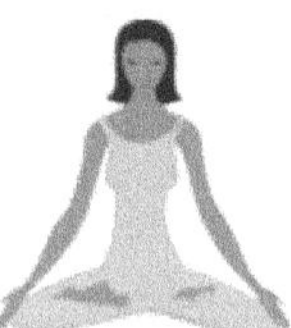

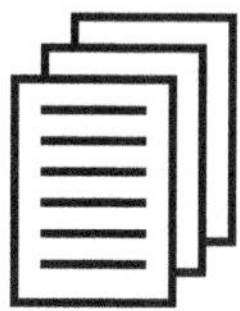

Managing hot flushes with relaxed breathing, thoughts and behaviour

Session 3

Professor Myra S Hunter and Dr Melanie Smith
Institute of Psychiatry, King's College London

Review the week

How are you getting on with the different aspects of the programme?

- Awareness of, and modification of your triggers
- Your individual stress reducing goals
- Relaxation practice

– in pairs discuss barriers you have encountered, and ways of overcoming them

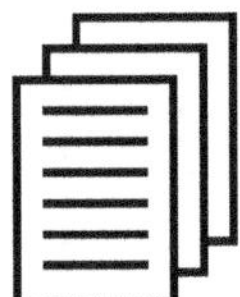

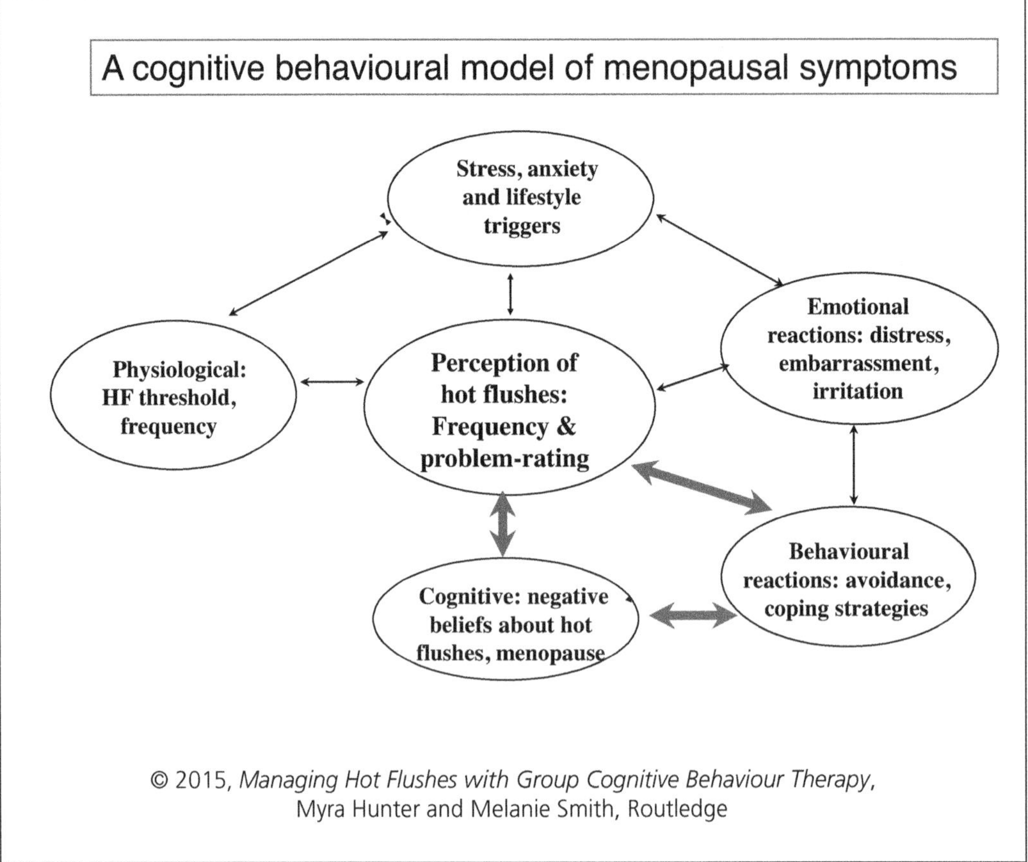
A cognitive behavioural model of menopausal symptoms
Stress, anxiety and lifestyle triggers
Physiological: HF threshold, frequency
Perception of hot flushes: Frequency & problem-rating
Emotional reactions: distress, embarrassment, irritation
Behavioural reactions: avoidance, coping strategies
Cognitive: negative beliefs about hot flushes, menopause
© 2015, Managing Hot Flushes with Group Cognitive Behaviour Therapy, Myra Hunter and Melanie Smith, Routledge

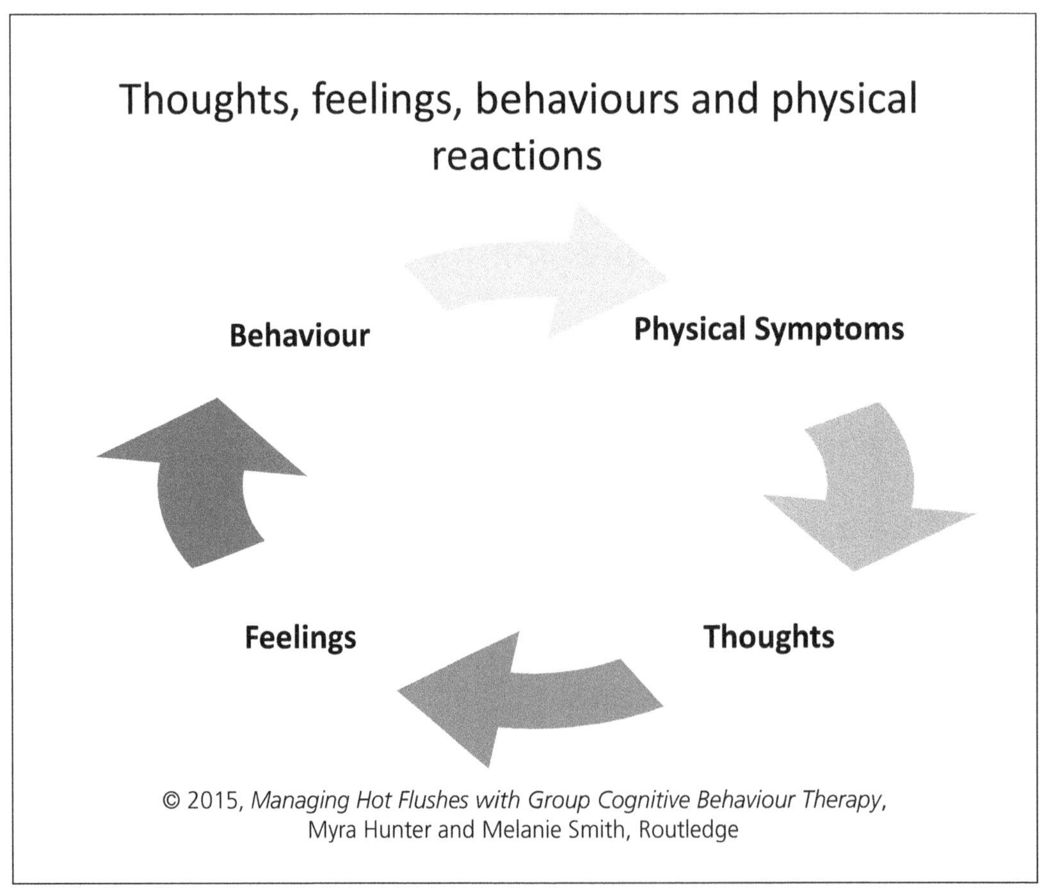
Thoughts, feelings, behaviours and physical reactions
Behaviour
Physical Symptoms
Feelings
Thoughts
© 2015, Managing Hot Flushes with Group Cognitive Behaviour Therapy, Myra Hunter and Melanie Smith, Routledge

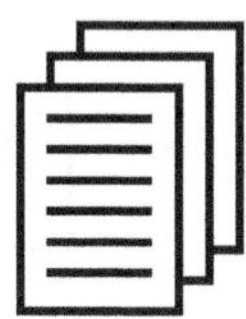

Thoughts, feelings, behaviours and physical reactions to hot flushes

Behaviour
Avoid situations, hide face, use fan,
Open windows, stop what I'm doing until it passes

Physical Symptoms
Heat, sweaty, palpitations, red face,
Breathless, nausea, tingling

Thoughts
People will think something is wrong
My body is letting me down
I look like a bag lady
Not another one!
I can't cope!

Feelings
Embarrassed, ashamed, anxious,
angry, trapped, frustrated,
out of control

Thoughts about hot flushes

- Thoughts are not facts and are one perspective on the situation
- Anxious thinking leads to feelings of anxiety
- Anxious thoughts about hot flushes may stem from:
  - Beliefs about the menopause/menopausal symptoms
  - Beliefs about yourself
  - Beliefs about the reactions of others
  - Beliefs about the future (expectations)
- Thinking patterns can influence coping

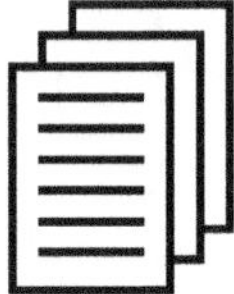

The role of thoughts on hot flushes

- Main types of worries around hot flushes and night sweats are:
  - Social embarrassment (especially around men or at work)
  - Lack of control
  - Worries about disrupted sleep
- Compared with women with low distress, women with the high levels of distress in reaction to hot flushes:
  - Tend to **catastrophise** about the hot flush (This is out of control, I can't cope with this)
  - They are more **self critical** within the situation, especially about their appearance e.g. dirty, smelly
  - Report more physical sensation (their attention focused only on flush)

Social situations

- When we feel self conscious in social situations we:
  - focus our attention inwards 'shine the spotlight on ourselves and imagine what others may see' (known as 'the observer perspective') which makes embarrassment worse
  - We tend to ignore EVERYTHING ELSE about the situation and focus only on ourselves which makes the flush seem more important than it is
- Embarrassment and shame arise from assumptions that others will be making negative judgements (mindreading)
  - These assumptions can arise from own negative views of self and menopause
- What do you assume others are thinking when you have a hot flush? (be aware of 'mindreading')
- Are you ignoring other information within the situation?

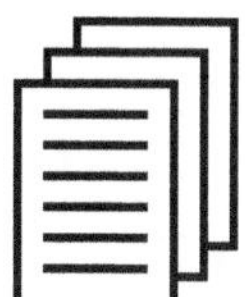

Supporting yourself in social situations

- Survey results – research shows that people:
  - Have a wide range of perceptions about possible causes of hot flushes
  - Do not tend to make any negative judgements
  - Feel concern/consideration for person having hot flushes
- Be aware of thinking patterns
  - Mindreading – how do you really know what someone else is definitely thinking? What else might they be thinking about?
  - Are you ignoring everything else about the situation and making the flush the focus?
- What would a calm/caring friend say to you – Develop compassionate approach to yourself
  - Would you talk to a friend in this way? What would you say to them to get them through the situation?
- Shift your focus of attention to breathing or external aspect of situation (don't focus on yourself/the flush)

Worries about control and frequency of hot flushes

- Examples of Control Worries:
  - 'Not another one!' 'I can't cope' 'This will never end'
  - 'I will pass out/collapse/lose control'
- Anticipatory thoughts/predictions that increase anxiety
- Tendency towards catastrophising
- Result in anger, feeling overwhelmed, anxiety, frustration, hopelessness
- Aim to develop *tolerance* of frustration caused by hot flush – pause and choose how to respond to increase control over hot flushes
  - Aim is to develop an attitude of *calm acceptance* rather than engaging with angry/irritable thoughts

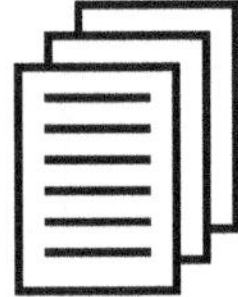

Enhancing sense of control

- Important to try to:
  - Develop an attitude of calm acceptance
  - Use paced breathing at the onset of a flush (helps to switch your attention to your breathing rather than the discomfort)
  - Identify catastrophising thoughts and deal with each flush one at a time
  - Letting the flush flow over you
- Enhance your sense of control through:
  - Understanding hot flushes
  - Checking your expectations
  - Behavioural response: Deep breath in, relax shoulders, supportive self statement and paced breathing
  - Managing stress

Helpful and unhelpful thoughts

UNHELPFUL THOUGHTS	MORE HELPFUL THOUGHTS
'Oh no I can't cope'	'Let's see how well I can deal with this one'
'Everyone's looking at me'	'I will notice my flushes more than other people'
'I am out of control	'There are things I can do to control them'
'Hot flushes are bad for my health'	'There's no evidence that this is the case – most women have them'
'I'm ashamed when I have hot flushes'	'Hot flushes are part of life'
'They will go on forever'	'They will gradually reduce over time'
'I don't want people to know that I'm going through the menopause'	'Menopause is a normal part of life that I shouldn't be ashamed of'

What would YOU think about someone else with hot flushes?

Group task

- Use the worksheet to identify thoughts if you need extra help
- Are these thoughts helping you to cope or not? Is there another way of thinking about the situation (e.g. from a friend's perspective?)
- Generate calm and helpful thoughts
- Feed back to group
- Practise as homework
  What is a more helpful way of thinking in this situation?

Behavioural responses to hot flushes

- What do you normally do?
- What is helpful or unhelpful?

  Brainstorm
- Practical changes that you can make?
- Addressing the key problem – AVOIDANCE
  - Short term benefit versus longer term loss!

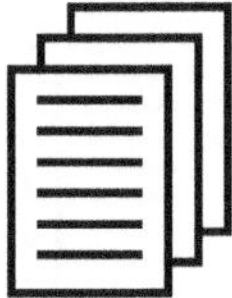

Behavioural responses: what helps?

- Cool down with sips of water, for example, wearing layers
- Try not to rush out of social situations
  - Humour?
  - Comment on it? Talk about it?
- Try not to avoid doing things that you would usually enjoy
- Deep breath – Flow over – Breath – Refocus

Applying relaxation and paced breathing

- Practise relaxation every day, continue stress reducing goals and pace activities to avoid rushing
- At the onset of a flush let your shoulders relax, breathe slowly from your stomach and concentrate on your breathing – let the flush flow over you as you relax

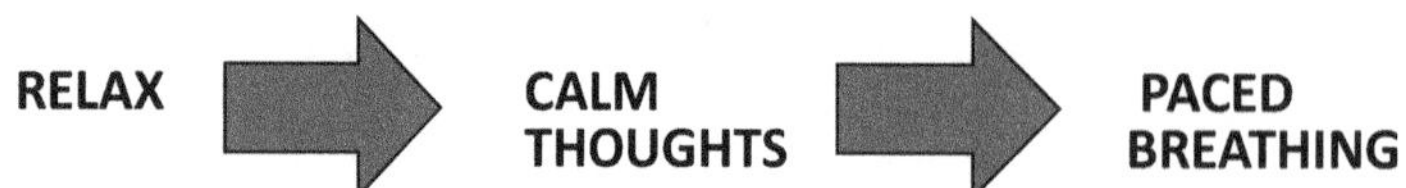

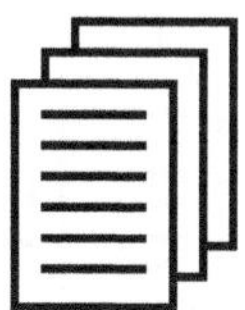

Homework

- Practise relaxation and *paced breathing at onset of hot flushes*, at specified times during the day and during stressful situations.
- Continue stress/wellbeing goals, which can be added to and modified each week.
- Look out for thinking during hot flushes and practise calm cognitive and behavioural responses.
- Complete sleep diary (a couple of nights) for next week's session.

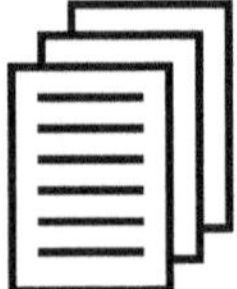

Managing night sweats and improving sleep (part one)

Session 4

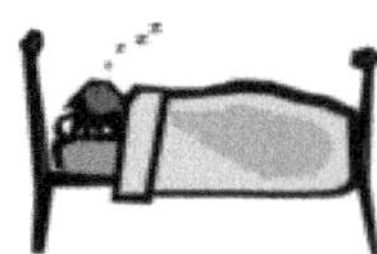

Professor Myra S Hunter and Dr Melanie Smith
Institute of Psychiatry, King's College London

Review the week

- How are you getting on with the different aspects of the programme?
  - Relaxation and paced breathing
  - Your individual stress reducing goals
  - Awareness and modification of your triggers
  - Identifying and modifying your thoughts at the time of a flush?
  - Using calming thoughts and relaxed breathing at the onset of a hot flush?
- In pairs discuss barriers you have encountered, and ways of overcoming them

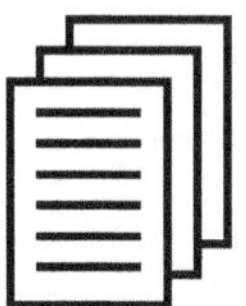

This session we will:

- Find out about improving sleep generally
- Establish the main ways night sweats affect our sleep patterns

NEXT WEEK

- Consider the influence that thinking and behaviour has on our sleep, and discuss what we can do to improve it
- Look at managing night sweats

What are your experiences of night sweats?

- Is there anything that you have noticed or that has particularly struck you from filling in your sleep diaries?
- How do night sweats affect your sleep?
- What do you do to manage them?
- Any impact on daytime tiredness?
- How do you cope?

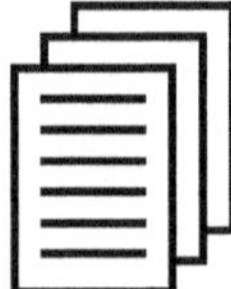

What can we do to manage night sweats and disrupted sleep?

- Get into better sleeping *habits* generally by making minor changes to our environment and sleep behaviour

- Reduce the stress of night sweats by:
  - Minimising activities other than sleep in the bedroom
  - Not restricting daytime activities due to night sweats
  - Using *routine* and *automatic* responses to night sweats to help you to manage night-time wakening (next week)
  - Managing our worries about night sweats and sleep doing some thought work (next week)

Sleep chart

Sleep enables cellular restoration – much brain activity in REM sleep and muscle repair activity in non REM

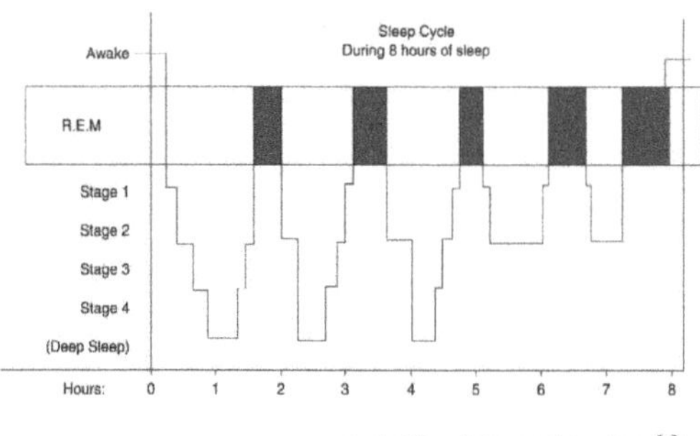

- Approximately 4–5 sleep cycles a night (each average 90–110 mins)
- Deep sleep (stages 3 and 4) occurs in the first half of the night (lack of this sleep relates to day time signs of tiredness)
- Night sweats more likely to wake you during lighter sleep
- Waking 1–3 times per night is normal

However,

- There is little evidence that poor sleep causes ill health (the body naturally goes to the stage most needed)
- Amount of sleep needed depends on: age, the individual, etc.
- Optimal average of 6–8 hrs a night. Quality more important than quantity
- It is normal to wake up, and after a poor night's sleep, we often seem to perform as well as usual – 'Good Enough Sleep'
- Stress and unhelpful beliefs about not sleeping are often the key problem

Thinking about sleep

Because sleep is a different 'state of awareness', our judgements are not always accurate about how long we sleep.

From recent research we know that most people:
- underestimate how much sleep they get, and
- overestimate the time it takes them to get to sleep

Studies have also shown that if we learn that we tend to make this misjudgement, i.e. sleep problem isn't as bad as we had thought, then we tend to worry less and sleep better.

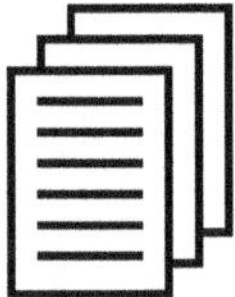

Developing better sleeping habits
Lifestyle and environmental factors

✧ Limit caffeine and alcohol

✧ Manage diet and exercise

✧ In the bedroom, try to reduce noise, reduce light, keep room temperature fairly cool

✧ Make your bed comfortable – is your mattress comfortable?

Developing better sleeping habits
Associating bed with sleep

✓ *Develop a strong positive association between sleep and your bed:*

✓ Only use your *bed for sleeping*

✓ Lie down in bed only when you feel *sleepy*

✓ If you're *awake* in bed for 15 minutes get up

✓ No napping *(if you must nap: do so before 3pm, no more than 1 hour!)*

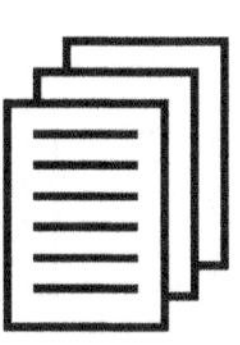

Developing better sleeping habits

Develop a good bedtime 'wind-down' routine

- Start to wind-down 60–90 minutes before going to bed using relaxing activities (e.g. bath)
- Include relaxation skills; full body relaxation or paced breathing
  - Learning to relax is a skill. It takes practice and it can take a while to learn to do it well
  - Relaxation and paced breathing can be practised as an automatic response for if you are woken by night sweats
  - Avoid clockwatching if you wake in the night as it increases anxiety

Developing better sleeping habits

Sleep scheduling

✓ Keep your sleep times as regular as possible

✓ Avoid going to bed too early to compensate for bad nights sleep

✓ Don't lie in – if you're awake, get up!

✓ Helps body's natural circadian rhythm to regulate so more likely to sleep once in bed

BED TIME (light off)	11.00pm
GETTING UP TIME	6.00am
TOTAL SLEEP TIME	7.00 hrs

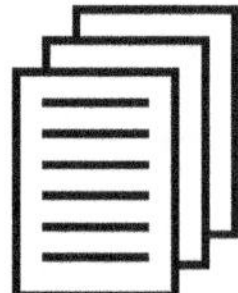

Developing better sleeping habits: *Managing daytime tiredness*

- It is important to try and continue with your day as planned.
- Avoid limiting activities
  - Limiting activities leads to low mood and increased levels of tiredness
  - Focuses your attention on your missing sleep ↑ preoccupation
- Continuing as normal and generating energy
  - Provides a distraction and can take your mind off feeling tired
  - It is helpful to try pacing your activities to avoid a 'boom and bust' cycle
  - Use energy generating activities rather than resting when feeling fatigued (e.g. running upstairs, 10 minutes fresh air, phone a friend)
  - Use *relaxation* rather than naps to manage tension arising from tiredness
- If this seems counterintuitive, try doing both (resting versus generating activity). Rate your tiredness on both days

Homework

- Daily practice of brief relaxation at specified time plus using *paced breathing at onset of hot flushes* and during stressful situations.
- Continue stress reducing and wellbeing goals.
- Continue to practise calm cognitive and behavioural responses to hot flushes.
- Implement sleep goals for next session.

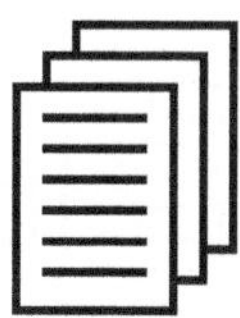

Managing sleep and night sweats (part two)

Session 5

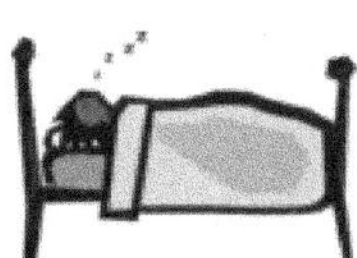

Professor Myra S Hunter and Dr Melanie Smith
Institute of Psychiatry, King's College London

Review the past week

How are you getting on with the different aspects of the programme?

- Relaxation and paced breathing and your stress/wellbeing goals, modification of your triggers
- Cognitive and behavioural strategies to manage hot flushes
- Using calming thoughts and relaxed breathing at the onset of a hot flush

In pairs discuss barriers you have encountered and ways of overcoming them

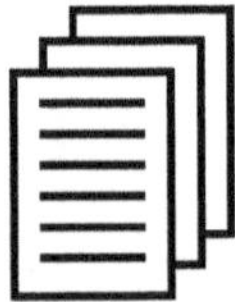

Group relaxation

- Practising relaxation and paced breathing at the onset of a flush
- Imagine that you are having a hot flush and breathe through it
- Continue to practise daily and if woken at night

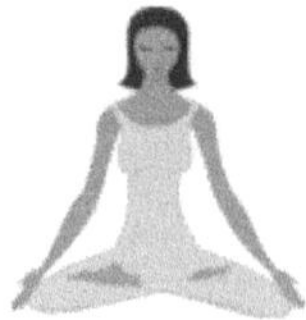

Night sweats and thoughts

Consider the following...

- What runs through your mind when you can't sleep?
- What runs through your mind the next day?
- How do you feel?

Night sweats and thoughts

Thought patterns that can disrupt sleep include...

- Worries carried over from the day
- Worrying about worrying
- Worries about not being able to sleep at night

Thinking about night sweats and sleep

- Using your knowledge about sleep from earlier in the session, can you come up with some alternative calmer thoughts to replace your stressful thoughts?
- Remembering:
  - 6–8 hours is adequate
  - Sleep onset and awareness
    - Tendency to overestimate time awake
    - Tendency to overestimate time getting to sleep
  - Impact of thinking when evaluating daytime tiredness

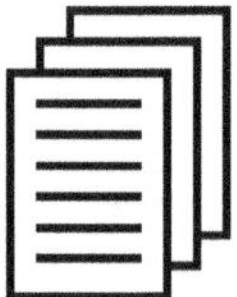

Thoughts about sleep

Less helpful thoughts:

Thinking catastrophic thoughts about the next day can lead to more worry

'I will be absolutely useless at work tomorrow!'

'If I have night sweats I'll feel terrible all day'

'I will look ten years older after having no sleep'

These thoughts are extreme (black and white thinking), with no middle ground, and they will have a negative impact on your emotional state

More helpful thoughts:

'I can get on with usual things even if I have had a bad night's sleep'

'Sleep problems are not dangerous or bad for me'

These thoughts provide a much more realistic appraisal of the situation

Your beliefs about sleep are important

Some useful *beliefs* are:

- Even if woken up at night, I can usually do what I need to the next day
- Having realistic expectations e.g. everyone (especially those experiencing night sweats) will have a poor night's sleep occasionally
- Recognise that not feeling completely rested some days is normal, EVEN AFTER a good night's sleep
- Most people feel tired when they first wake up

Have you changed any of your beliefs about sleep and night sweats since starting this work?

How to deal with stress that keeps you awake

If you are worrying about something separate to sleep and night sweats:

- ✓ Allow thoughts to flow over you, to come and go, e.g. like trains passing through a station
- ✓ Paced breathing to reduce arousal levels!
- ✓ Think about a relaxing scene and focus on breathing
- ✓ Establish 'Worry Time' – deal with worrisome thoughts by making time in the day to focus on the concern, using problem-solving to find solutions while awake

Also, remember that there are helpful things that you can *do*:

- ✓ Wind-down routine
- ✓ Keep your sleep schedule as regular as you are able
- ✓ Cut out negative lifestyle influences from your life and bedroom area
- ✓ Avoid spending too much time in bed
- ✓ Use relaxation and relaxing scenes to calm your mind and body
- ✓ Avoid napping in the daytime
- ✓ Avoid cancelling daytime activities

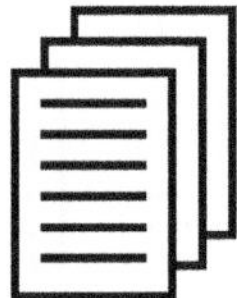

Calmly responding to night sweats

- Calmly get up and do what you need to in order to cool down; keep lights dimmed
- Watch your thoughts while doing this – if they have become worried/anxious remember it is a thought rather than a FACT
- Once you have cooled off, get back into bed and practise relaxation and paced breathing
- Watch thoughts – don't engage with them, return the focus of your attention to your breathing

Summary of sleep advice

Behaviour:

Manage unhelpful environmental and lifestyle factors. Maintain a regular sleep pattern

Thinking:

Manage worrying thoughts – about various concerns you have + about sleep itself

Feelings and physical stress:

Practice relaxation and paced breathing to reduce overall stress by providing balance to busy lives, to manage hot flushes/night sweats and to induce sleepiness when required

Develop a good bedtime wind-down routine

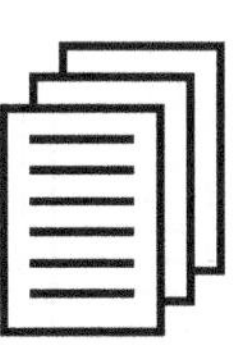

Sleep action plan

- From what you have heard, and given your own specific situation, what can you do to start improving your sleep?

- Write down two things that you want to do and which you have a good chance (75%) of doing over the next week

- Are there any ways you can manage worrying thoughts about sleep or stress?

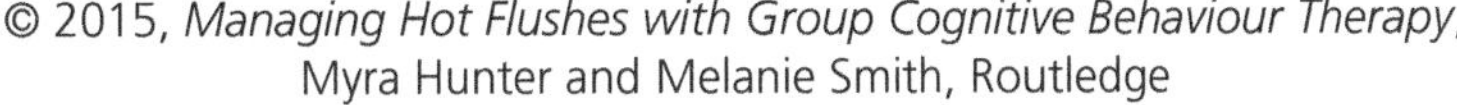

Homework

✓ Implement a sleep action plan to include behavioural work from last week as well as cognitive work from this week.

✓ Continue with wellbeing goals and precipitant modification.

✓ Continue using breathing/relaxation if stressed and at times during the day.

✓ Continue to apply calming thoughts and paced breathing automatically at the onset of hot flushes and night sweats.

© 2015, *Managing Hot Flushes with Group Cognitive Behaviour Therapy*, Myra Hunter and Melanie Smith, Routledge

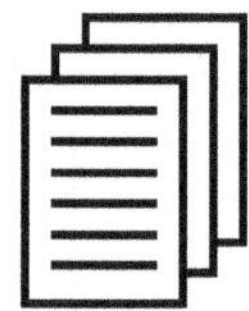

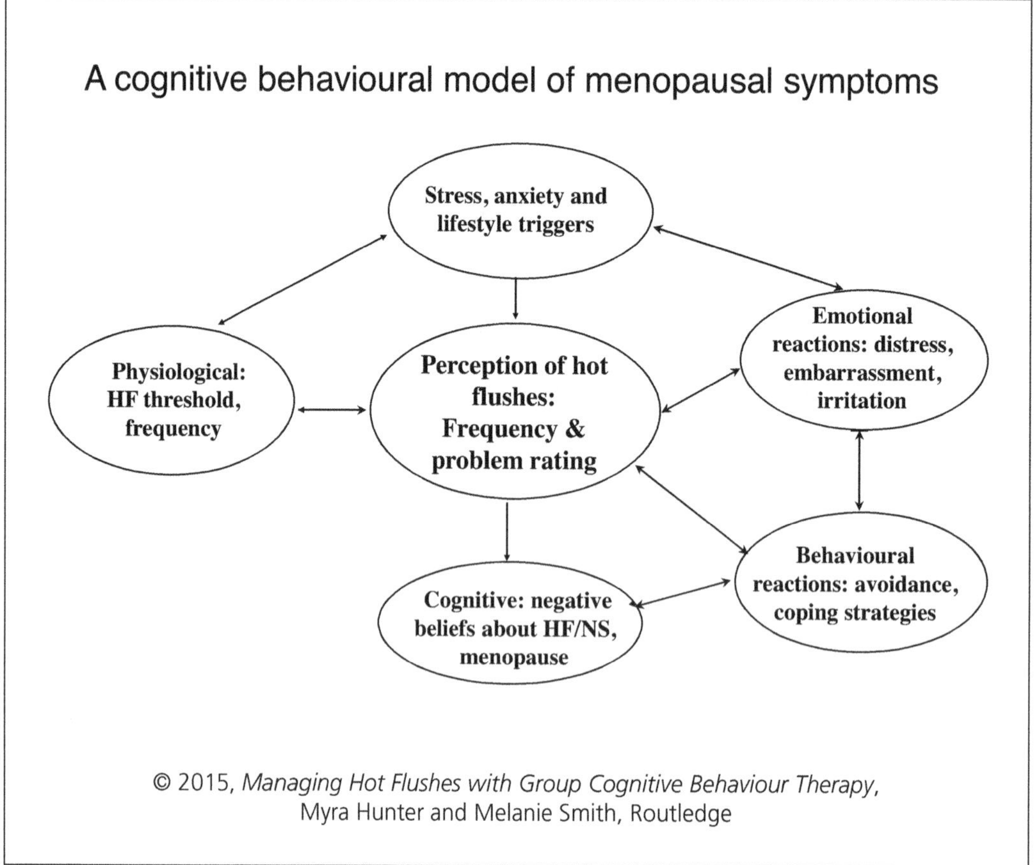
A cognitive behavioural model of menopausal symptoms
Stress, anxiety and lifestyle triggers
Physiological: HF threshold, frequency
Perception of hot flushes: Frequency & problem rating
Emotional reactions: distress, embarrassment, irritation
Behavioural reactions: avoidance, coping strategies
Cognitive: negative beliefs about HF/NS, menopause

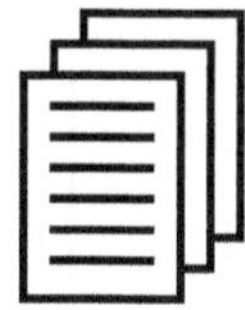

Managing hot flushes and night sweats: review

Session 6

Professor Myra S Hunter and Dr Melanie Smith
Institute of Psychiatry, King's College London

Today's session

- Review and acknowledge progress so far
- Work out how to:
  - keep it going
  - take it forward
- Brief review of what we've learnt
- Develop maintenance plans
- Open discussion

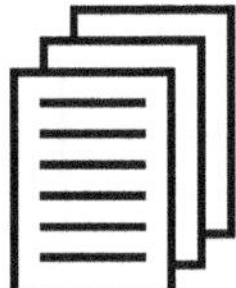

How did you get on with your homework?

Developing new habits...

- Sleeping environment?
- Bedtime routine?
- Relaxation response?
- Linking bed and sleep?
- Limiting time in bed?
- Managing daytime tiredness?
- Managing thoughts around night sweats and sleep?

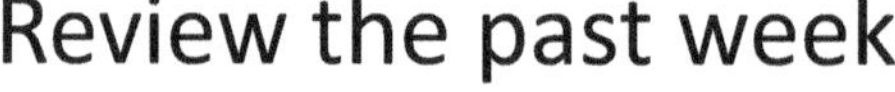

Review the past week

How are you getting on with the different aspects of the programme?

- Relaxation and paced breathing
- Your individual stress reducing goals
- Awareness and modification of your triggers
- Identifying and modifying thoughts at time of a hot flush
- Using calming thoughts and relaxed breathing at the onset of a hot flush

In pairs discuss progress and any barriers you have encountered and ways of overcoming them

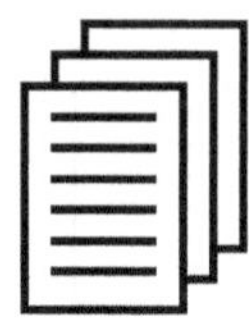

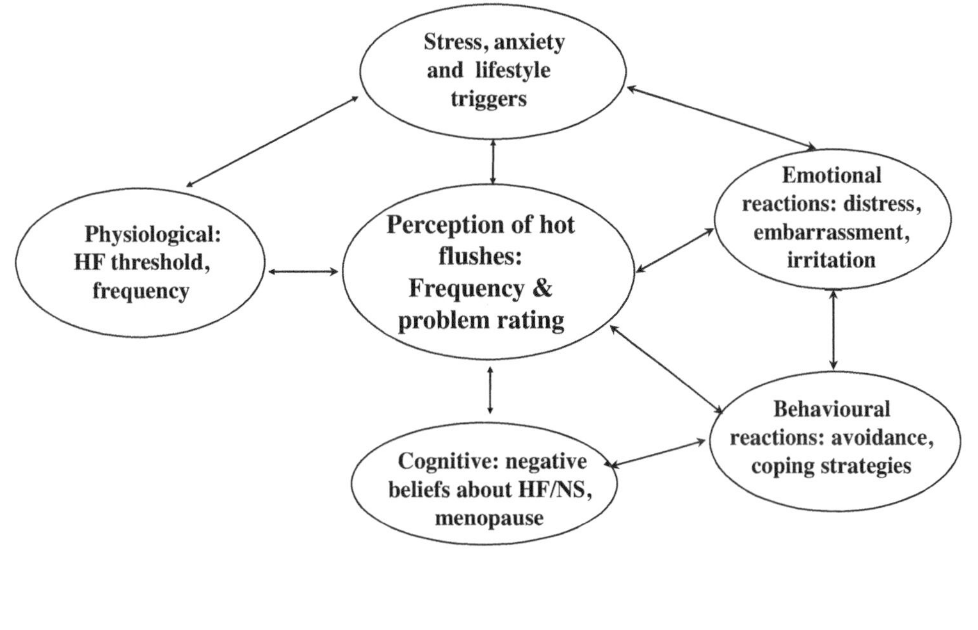

Managing hot flushes and night sweats

- Identifying and modifying precipitants
- Relaxation and paced breathing
- Stress management and lifestyle changes
- Problem-solving
- Pacing activities and exercise
- Hot flushes: modifying thoughts and behaviours
- Practising breathing and calm thoughts for hot flushes
- Dealing with social situations
- Night sweats and sleep: modifying thoughts and behaviours

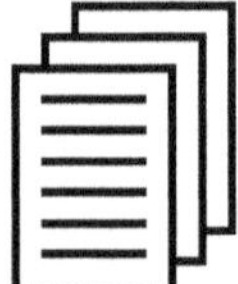

Develop a maintenance plan...

Identify 2–3 concrete goals

but first consider the following...

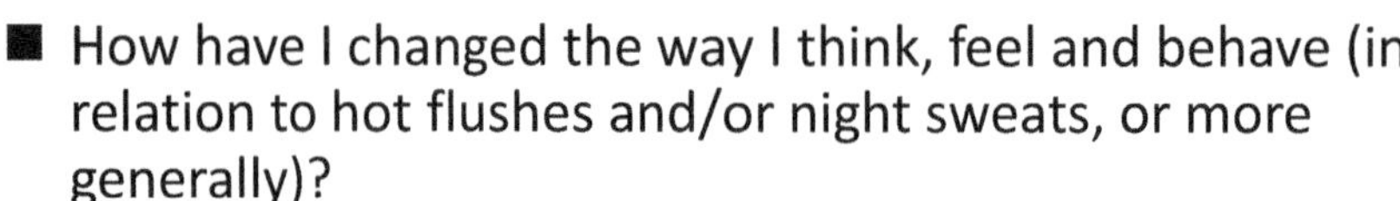

- How have I changed the way I think, feel and behave (in relation to hot flushes and/or night sweats, or more generally)?
- What might be a future barrier which may get in the way of me keeping up changes?
- How will I know I'm having a setback? (Think of changes in feelings, behaviours, or thoughts which may be a sign that changes aren't maintained)
- If I do have a setback, what can I do about it?

General advice: maintaining changes

- Make realistic plans to help manage your hot flushes and night sweats over the coming weeks and months
- They may vary with what is happening in your life
- Use them to take stock and to reduce stress and to use the strategies that help you
- If you anticipate stress or problems then use helpful strategies more during these times
- Remember that you share this experience with many other women

Group discussion

Potential topics for open discussion:

- Breast cancer – experience and treatments
- Adjustment across the menopause transition
- Sexuality and the menopause
- Body image and weight gain
- Memory
- Osteoporosis
- Managing pain
- Other?

Breast cancer – experience and treatments

- Anxieties about uncertainty, recurrence and follow-up appointments are common
- Cognitive reactions: thoughts can make one feel helpless or be overly pessimistic:

  ...if I don't know what's going to happen there's no point doing anything
- Behavioural reactions can include checking, avoidance, seeking reassurance
- Behavioural strategies such as activity scheduling can be helpful and it can help to have expectations that aren't overly negative, to be in control of some aspects of life, and to make use of social support
- Discuss how people generally deal with the uncertainties of life...
- You may also need to adapt and make changes to reduce demands on yourself following your illness/tiredness following treatment – be aware of extreme, or black and white, thinking about this.

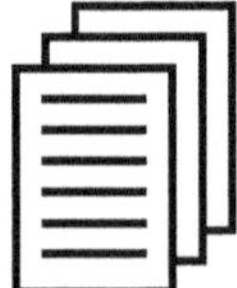

The menopause transition

- Menopause can be a time of transition and uncertainty
- Unfamiliar process leading to reflection about the past and possibly anxiety about the future
- Other different transitional phases in life you have managed?

The menopause transition: helpful approaches

- Knowing this is a normal stage of life (including feelings)
- Retain hope and confidence that you will navigate through
- Looking after yourself
- Schedule in pleasant activities and time for yourself
- Using stress management techniques
- Be in a state of readiness, being open to new experiences to fill any empty spaces that may arise
- Are there any things you used to enjoy doing that you could pick up again now – pleasure or achievement?

Sexuality and the menopause

- Women often report a decrease in sexual interest during menopause and with age but there are considerable differences between women

- Can be accompanied by other symptoms:
  - Vaginal dryness
  - Poor body image
  - Pain during intercourse

- Decrease in libido is due to a variety of factors
  - Beliefs and expectations about ageing and sexuality
  - Stress and overwork
  - Fatigue from night sweats and sleep disruption
  - Relationship conflict/tension
  - Oestrogen reduction, causing vaginal dryness
  - Health issues

Sexuality

- Psychological approaches
  - Managing stress
  - Identifying and addressing unhelpful beliefs about ageing and sexuality
  - Communicating with partner/having a discussion about any worries
  - Using relaxation
- Physiological approaches
  - Using lubricants
  - Finding alternatives to intercourse for physical intimacy
  - Massage
  - Changing position
  - Exercise (increases sex drive)
  - Pelvic floor exercises

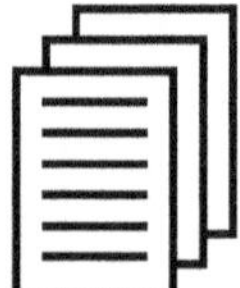

Body image and weight gain

- Reduced oestrogen levels can lead to redistribution of fat to stomach, but not necessarily weight increase
- Illness such as breast cancer can lead to weight gain too
- There is evidence suggesting that weight loss, using a healthy diet and exercise, can lead to improvements in quality of life and also to improvements in hot flushes (Davis et al. 2012).
- How can you fit a sensible diet and some exercise into your day? (e.g. gardening, brisk walks, daily tasks?)

Memory

- Limited evidence that memory is affected solely by menopause – both men and women show evidence of age related memory decline.
- Other factors are also important: stress, psychological factors such as low mood, anxiety.
- Doing one thing at a time helps to improve attention and memory.
- If you want to remember something specific linking it to a mental image can be helpful.
- Don’t worry too much or try too hard.

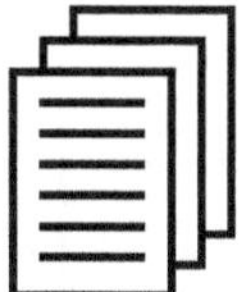

Osteoporosis

- Low bone mass susceptible to fractures
- Oestrogen helps to maintain bone mass
- Risk factors
  - Being female – less dense bone mass
  - Genetic factors
  - Early menopause (< 45 years old)
  - Smoking
  - 14 units of alcohol + per week
  - Low calcium diet
  - Lack of weight bearing exercise

Osteoporosis management and prevention

- Diet
  - 700mg of calcium daily (equivalent to a pint of semi skimmed milk)
  - Low fat dairy products
  - Oily fish, green leafy veg, bread, cereals
  - Needs vit D to absorb; oily fish, margarine, eggs and sun!
  - 5 fruit and veg per day to ensure mineral intake

- Reduce caffeine intake as this affects absorption
- Stop smoking
- Reduce alcohol intake to less than 14 units per week
- Supplements? See GP

- Weight bearing exercise:
  - Walking, jogging, dancing, running, tennis, skipping, aerobics, any extra as part of daily routine e.g. walk to bus stop etc.

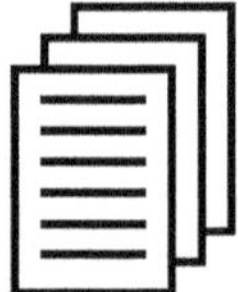

Managing pain

- Experience of pain influenced by range of factors:
  - Anxiety, depression, stress, sleep difficulties
- Thinking styles (e.g. catastrophising) and attention focus may lead to a vicious cycle

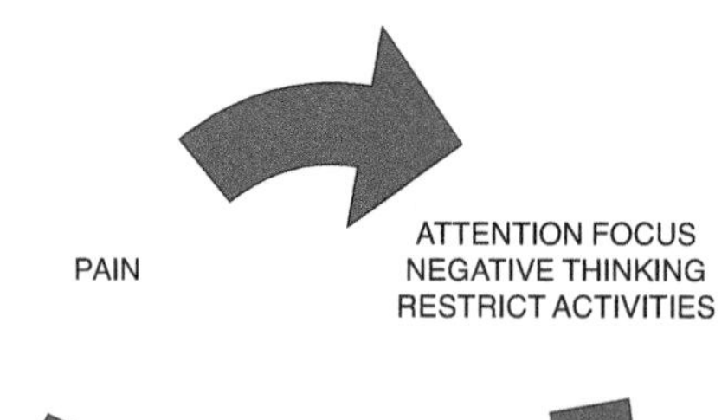

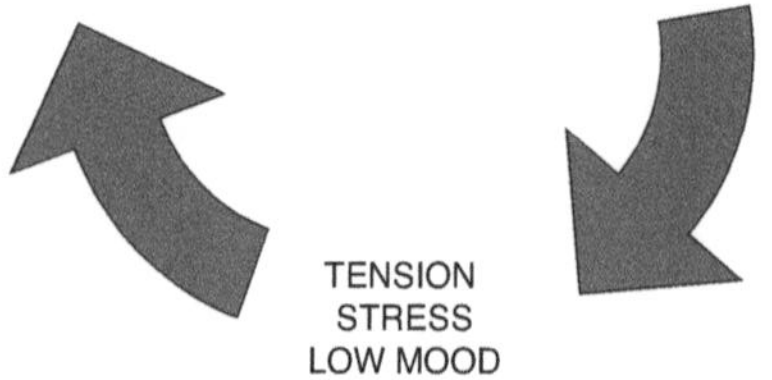

Managing pain

- Using relaxation and calm breathing
- Pacing activities:
  - Breaking down into manageable chunks
  - Reducing unnecessary demands/pressure
  - Maintaining activity rather than reducing
- Scheduling pleasant activities
- Checking thinking for catastrophising and negative predictions (e.g 'this will never end' or 'it will get worse')
- Checking attention focus
- Use the strategies above but ask for help if/when you need to.

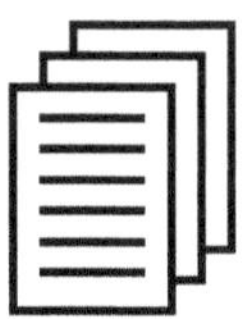

Group relaxation

- Practising relaxation and paced breathing when feeling signs of stress and at the onset of a flush
- Continue to practise and integrate into daily life

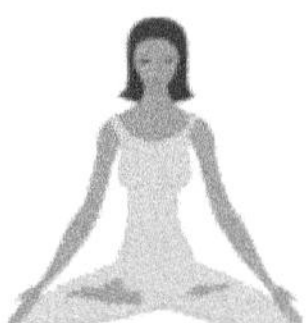

And finally....

- Goodbyes

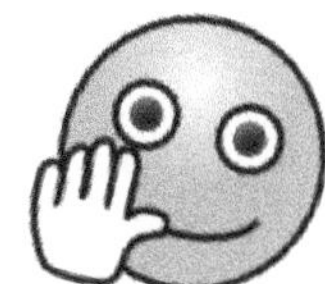

- Complete Hot Flush Rating Scale.

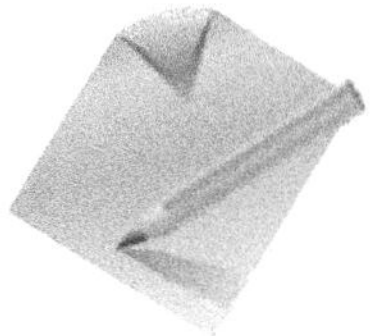

© 2015, *Managing Hot Flushes with Group Cognitive Behaviour Therapy*, Myra Hunter and Melanie Smith, Routledge

Resources

MENOPAUSE

International Menopause Society

The aims of the IMS are to promote knowledge, study and research on all aspects of ageing in men and women; to organise, prepare, hold and participate in international meetings and congresses on menopause and to encourage the interchange of research plans and experience between individual members.

www.imsociety.org
Ms Lee Tomkins
IMS Executive Director
PO Box 98
Camborne
Cornwall, UK TR14 4BQ
Tel: +44 (0) 1209 711 054
Email: leetomkinsims@btinternet.com

British Menopause Society

The British Menopause Society (BMS) is a registered charity and multidisciplinary society for women seeking information and advice as well as nurses and doctors and other health professionals. Although primarily a professional organisation, the BMS website includes information aimed at the general public, including a number of fact sheets on various aspects of the menopause.

www.thebms.org.uk
British Menopause Society
4–6 Eton Place
Marlow
Buckinghamshire, UK SL7 2QA
Tel: + 44 (0) 1628 890199
Fax: + 44 (0) 1628 474042

North American Menopause Society

The North American Menopause Society (NAMS) is a leading non-profit organisation dedicated to promoting the health and quality of life of women during midlife and beyond through an understanding of menopause and healthy ageing. Its multidisciplinary membership includes clinical and basic science experts from medicine, nursing, sociology, psychology, nutrition, anthropology, epidemiology, pharmacy, and education and enables NAMS to provide balanced information. Includes sections for health professionals as well as women experiencing menopause. It publishes the journal *Menopause Management*.

www.menopause.org
5900 Landerbrook Drive
Suite 390
Mayfield Heights, OH 44124, USA
Tel: + 1 440 442 7550
Email: info@menopause.org

Menopause Exchange (newsletter and website)

The Menopause Exchange gives independent advice and is not sponsored by commercial organisations. It provides information on a range of topics, including menopausal symptoms, osteoporosis, self-help measures, HRT, alternatives to HRT and products. Its 'Ask the Experts' panel includes many of the UK's top health care professionals working in the field of the menopause. The site features a blog and online articles.

www.menopause-exchange.co.uk
The Menopause Exchange
PO Box 205
Bushey, Herts, UK WD23 1ZS
Tel: + 44 (0) 20 8420 7245
Fax: +44 (0) 20 8954 2783
Email: info@menopause-exchange.co.uk

Menopause Support

A not-for-profit enterprise helping women to share remedies, advice and information based on their own experience. Its website includes a blog and suggestions for dietary change. It also offers workshops and one-to-one telephone advice as well as Facebook and Twitter accounts.

www.menopausesupport.org.uk
Tel: +44 (0) 1392 876122
Email: info@menopausesupport.org.uk

Menopause Matters

An independent website providing up-to-date, accurate information about the menopause, menopausal symptoms and treatment options. It offers information on what happens leading up to, during and after the menopause, what the consequences can be, what you can do to help and what treatments are available. You can keep in touch via its Facebook and Twitter accounts.

www.menopausematters.co.uk

The Daisy Network

The Daisy Network Premature Menopause Support Group is a registered UK charity for women who have experienced a premature menopause. It is a not-for-profit organisation. The website provides information about premature menopause and the issues around it.

www.daisynetwork.org.uk
The Daisy Network
PO Box 183
Rossendale, Lancashire, UK BB4 6WZ

Fertility Friends

Fertility Friends is a web-based information and support community. Its message boards allow you to ask a nurse and other relevant professionals questions, or to chat with other people affected by infertility.

www.fertilityfriends.co.uk

GENERAL WOMEN'S HEALTH AND WELLBEING

Women's Health Concern

Women's Health Concern is the UK's leading charity providing help and advice to women on a wide variety of health, wellbeing and lifestyle concerns, to enable them to work in partnership with their own medical practitioners. Information is offered by telephone, email, in print, online and through conferences, seminars and symposia.

www.womens-health-concern.org
4–6 Eton Place
Marlow, Bucks, UK SL7 2QA
Tel (office): +44 (0) 1628 478 473
Advice line: + 44 (0) 845 123231

Women's Health London

Telephone helpline offering assistance on various aspects of women's health.

www.womenshealthlondon.org.uk.
52 Featherstone Street
London EC1Y 8RT
Helpline: +44 (0) 845 125 5254
Tel: +44 (0) 20 7251 6333
Fax: +44 (0) 20 7250 4152
Email: health@womenshealthlondon.org.uk

Women's Health

Online site offering information and forums around all aspects of women's health including many aspects of menopause.

www.womens-health.co.uk

NHS Live Well

An NHS website offering health and wellbeing advice including real stories and online assessment tools for all ages, but with specific sections for women aged 40–60 and 60+, including many aspects of menopause as well as keeping healthy.

www.nhs.uk/LiveWell/Women4060/Pages/Women4060home.aspx

Breast Cancer Care

This charity offers information and emotional and practical support to people affected by breast cancer.

www.breastcancercare.org.uk
5–13 Great Suffolk Street
London SE1 0NS
Helpline: +44 (0) 808 800 6000
Email: info@breastcancercare.org.uk
General enquiries switchboard: +44 (0) 845 092 0800

Cancer Research UK

Its website provides information about all types of cancer, spotting early symptoms, and the emotional consequences of a cancer diagnosis. Also provided are an e-newsletter, Twitter posts, blogs and podcasts. The charity funds research into cancer and provides telephone helpline support.

www.cancerresearchuk.org
Angel Building
407 St John Street
London EC1V 4AD
Tel (Supporter Services): +44 (0) 300 123 1022
Tel (Switchboard): +44 (0) 20 7242 0200

Breast Cancer Campaign

Provides information on coping with breast cancer as well as blogs, a Facebook page and funding into breast cancer research. It runs the 'pink campaign' to raise awareness of breast cancer.

www.breastcancercampaign.org
Clifton Centre
110 Clifton Street
London EC2A 4HT
Tel: +44 (0) 20 7749 4114

Macmillan Cancer Support

Provides practical, medical and financial support and campaigns for better cancer care via its website and local groups. It also offers an online community for people diagnosed with cancer and for carers.

www.macmillan.org.uk
89 Albert Embankment
London SE1 7UQ
Helpline: + 44 (0) 808 808 00 00

National Osteoporosis Society

Offers information about osteoporosis through a range of booklets, magazines, telephone helpline and regional support groups.

www.nos.org.uk
Camerton
Bath BA2 0PJ
Tel: +44 (0) 1761 471771 or +44 (0) 845 130 3076
Email: info@nos.org.uk

MENTAL HEALTH AND SELF-HELP TOOLS

Increasing Access to Psychological Therapy (IAPT) services

For details of Increasing Access to Psychological Therapy (IAPT) services in your area, please go to www.nhs.uk/service-search/counselling-nhs-(iapt)-services/locationsearch/396 and enter your town/postcode. You can also contact your GP for a referral.

www.iapt.nhs.uk

Moodjuice

Moodjuice is an Internet site developed by Choose Life Falkirk and the Adult Clinical Psychology Service, NHS Forth Valley. The site is designed to offer information and advice to those experiencing troublesome thoughts, feelings and actions. From the site you are able to print off various self-help guides covering conditions such as depression, anxiety, stress, panic and sleep problems.

www.moodjuice.scot.nhs.uk/

Northumberland, Tyne and Wear NHS Foundation Trust

Northumberland, Tyne and Wear NHS Foundation Trust is one of the largest mental health and disability Trusts in England and provides downloadable CBT-based self-help guides for conditions including anxiety, panic, anger, obsessions and compulsions, and bereavement.

www.ntw.nhs.uk/pic/selfhelp

Royal College of Psychiatrists

Readable, user-friendly and accurate information about mental health problems, including signposting to relevant services.

www.rcpsych.ac.uk/expertadvice.aspx

Mind

Mind publishes information on many topics relating to mental health, grouped into seven broad categories: diagnoses and conditions, treatments, mental health statistics, support and social care, communities and social groups, and society and environment.

www.mind.org.uk/
PO Box 277
Manchester M60 3XN
Tel: +44 (0) 300 123 3393
Email: info@mind.org.uk

PSYCHOTHERAPY

British Psychological Society

The British Psychological Society is the representative body for psychology and psychologists in the UK. It is responsible for the development, promotion and application of psychology.

www.bps.org.uk/psychology-public/find-psychologist/find-psychologist
www.counselling.co.uk
1 Regent Place
Rugby, Warks, UK CV21 2PJ
Tel: +44 (0) 870 443 5252
Fax : +44 (0) 870 443 5160
Email: bac@bac.co.uk

British Association for Behavioural and Cognitive Psychotherapy

A lead organisation for CBT in the UK and Ireland. Its website includes a register of accredited CBT therapists.

www.babcp.com
Imperial House
Hornby Street
Bury, Lancashire, UK BL9 5BN
Tel: + 44 (0) 161 705 4304

The Samaritans

Helpline offering emotional support for anyone in a crisis.

www.samaritans.org.uk
10 The Grove
Slough, UK SL1 1QP
Helpline: +44 (0) 845 790 9090
Fax: + 44 (0) 1753 819 004
Email: jo@samaritans.org.uk

Turn2me

An online mental health community offering peer and professional support for people suffering from anxiety and depression, including online CBT tools, a blog, information articles, and podcasts.

www.turn2me.org
Turn2MeUK
1 Pendlebury
Hamworth
Bracknell, Berks, UK RG12 7RB

ANXIETY

No Panic

The National Organisation for Phobias, Anxiety, Neurosis, Information and Care. Its website has a range of downloadable information booklets.

www.nopanic.org.uk
Unit 3
Prospect House
Halesfield 22
Telford, Shrops TF7 4QX
Tel: + 44 (0) 1952 680460
Email: ceo@nopanic.org.uk

DEPRESSION

The Depression Alliance

The website contains information about the symptoms of depression, treatments for depression, as well as research, publications, campaigns, and local self-help groups.

www.depressionalliance.org/
20 Great Dover Street
London SE1 4LX
Email: information@depressionalliance.org

MISCELLANEOUS SUPPORT

Relate

Relationship counselling.
www.relate.org.uk
Premier House
Carolina Court
Lakeside
Doncaster DN4 5RA
Tel: 0300 100 1234

Carers UK

Information and advice on all aspects of caring.

www.carersuk.demon.co.uk
20–25 Glasshouse Yard
London EC1A 4JT
Carers' line: 0808 808 7777
Tel: +44 (0) 20 7490 8818
Fax: +44 (0) 20 7490 8824
Email: info@ukcarers.org

Careline

Telephone counselling on any issue.

Cardinal Heenan Centre
326 High Road
Ilford, Essex IG1 1QP
Helpline: +44 (0) 20 8514 1177
Office tel: +44 (0) 8514 5444
Fax: + 44 (0) 20 8478 7943
Email: careline@totalise.co.uk

Cruse Bereavement Care

Provides support services for people who have been bereaved.

www.crusebereavementcare.org.uk
126 Sheen Road
Richmond, Surrey TW9 1UR
Helpline: 0870 167 1677
Office tel: +44 (0) 20 8939 9530
Fax: + 44 (0) 20 8939 9530
Email: info@crusebereavementcare.org.uk

Divorce Support Group (DSG)

A professionally run organisation providing local support groups and individual support to help you cope with the emotional and psychological impact of your divorce or separation.

www.divorcesupportgroup.co.uk
Tel: + 44 (0) 844 800 90 98
Email: mail@divorcesupportgroup.co.uk

The Athena Network

A networking site for women, which aims to help members link up across a range of industry sectors.

www.theathenanetwork.co.uk
30 Northfield Gardens
Watford, Herts, UK WD24 7RE
Email: enquiries@theathenanetwork.co.uk

References

Andrikoula, M. and Prevelic, G. (2009) Menopausal hot flushes revisited. *Climacteric*, 12(1), 3–15.

Archer, D.F., Sturdee, D.W., Baber, R., de Villiers T.J., Pines, A., Freedman, R.R. et al. (2011) Menopausal hot flushes and night sweats: where are we now? *Climacteric*, 14(5), 515–28.

Avis, N.E., Zhao, X., Johannes, C., Ory, M., Brockwell, S. and Greendale, G. (2005) Correlates of sexual function among multi-ethnic middle-aged women: results from the Study of Women's Health Across the Nation (SWAN). *Menopause*, 12(4), 385–98.

Ayers, B. and Hunter, M.S. (2013) Health-related quality of life of women with menopausal hot flushes and night sweats. *Climacteric*, 16(2), 235.

Ayers, B., Forshaw, M. and Hunter, M.S. (2010) The impact of attitudes towards the menopause on women's symptom experience: A systematic review. *Maturitas*, 65(1), 28–36.

Ayers, B., Mann, E. and Hunter, M.S. (2011) A randomised controlled trial of a group and self help cognitive behavioural interventions for women who have menopausal symptoms MENOS 2. *British Medical Journal Open*. DOI: 10.1136/bmjopen-2010-000047.

Ayers, B., Smith, M., Hellier, J., Mann, E. and Hunter, M.S. (2012) Effectiveness of group and self-help cognitive behaviour therapy to reduce problematic menopausal hot flushes and night sweats (MENOS 2): a randomised controlled trial. *Menopause*, 19(7), 749–59.

Balabanovic, J., Ayers, B. and Hunter, M.S. (2012) An exploration of women's experiences of group cognitive behaviour therapy to treat breast cancer treatment-related hot flushes and night sweats: an interpretative phenomenological analysis. *Maturitas*, 72(3), 236–42.

Balabanovic, J., Ayers, B. and Hunter, M.S. (2013) Cognitive behaviour therapy for menopausal hot flushes and night sweats: a qualitative analysis of women's experiences of Group and Self-Help CBT. *Behavioural and Cognitive Psychotherapy*, 41(4), 441–57.

Beral, V. (2003) Breast cancer and hormone replacement therapy in the Million Women study. *Lancet*, 362(9382), 419–27.

Borrelli, F. and Ernst, E. (2010) Alternative and complementary therapies for the menopause. *Maturitas*, 66(4), 333–43.

Burger, H.G. (2006) Physiology and endocrinology of the menopause. *Medicine*, 34(1), 27–30.

Carmody, J.F., Crawford, S., Salmoirago- Blotcher, E., Leung, K., Churchill, L. and Olendzki, N. (2011) Mindfulness training for coping with hot flushes: results of a randomized trial. *Menopause*, 18(6), 611–20.

Carpenter, J., Johnson, D., Wagner, L. and Andrykowski, M. (2002) Hot flushes and related outcomes in breast cancer survivors and matched comparison women. *Oncology Nursing Forum*, 29(3), 16–25.

Carroll, D.G. (2006) Non-hormonal therapies for hot flushes in menopause. *American Family Physician*, 73(3), 457–64.

Chilcot, J., Norton, S. and Hunter, M.S. (2014) Cognitive behaviour therapy for menopausal symptoms following breast cancer treatment: who benefits and how does it work? *Maturitas* 78(1), 56–61.

Cioffi, D. (1991) Beyond attentional strategies: a cognitive perceptual model of somatic interpretation. *Psychological Bulletin*, 109(1), 25–41.

Col, N.F., Guthrie, J.R., Politi, M. and Dennerstein, L. (2009) Duration of vasomotor symptoms in middle aged women: a longitudinal study. *Menopause*, 16(3), 453–57.

Committee on Safety of Medicines. (2002) Safety update on long-term HRT. *Current Problems in Pharmacovigilance*, 28, 11–12.

Davis, S.R., Castelo-Branco, C., Chedraui, P., Lumsden, M.A., Nappi, R.E., Shah, D. et al. (2012) Understanding weight gain at menopause. *Climacteric*, 15(5), 419–29.

Dennerstein, L., Lehert, P. and Burger, H. (2005) The relative effects of hormones and relationship factors on sexual function of women through the natural menopausal transition. *Fertility and Sterility*, 84(10), 174–80.

Dennerstein, L., Guthrie, J.R., Clark, M., Lehert, P. and Henderson, V.W. (2004) A population-based study of depressed mood in middle-aged, Australian-born women. *Menopause*, 11(5), 563–68.

de Villiers, T.J., Gass, M.L.S., Haines, C.J., Hall, J.E., Lobo, R.A. et al. (2013). Global Consensus Statement on menopausal hormone therapy. *Climacteric*, 16 (2), 203–204.

Duijts, S.F.A., van Beurden, M., Oldenburg, H.S.A., Hunter, M.S., Kieffer, J.M., Stuiver, M.M. et al. (2012) Efficacy of cognitive behavioral therapy and physical exercise in alleviating treatment-induced menopausal symptoms in patients with breast cancer: results of a randomized, controlled, multicenter trial. *Journal of Clinical Oncology*, 30(33), 4124–33.

Espie, C.A. (2006) *Overcoming insomnia and sleep problems*. London, UK: Constable and Robinson.

Fenlon, D.R. and Rogers, A.E. (2007) The experience of hot flushes after breast cancer. *Cancer Nursing*, 30(4), 19–26.

Fenlon, D.R., Corner, J.L. and Haviland, J.S. (2008) A randomised trial of relaxation training to reduce hot flushes in women with primary breast cancer. *Journal of Pain and Symptom Management*, 35(4), 397–405.

Ferrie, J.E., Shipley, M.J, and Marmot, M.G (2007) A prospective study of change in sleep duration: associations with mortality I the Whitehall II Cohort. *Sleep*, 30(12), 1658–66.

Flint, M. (1975) The menopause; reward or punishment? *Psychosomatics*, 16(4), 161–63.

Ford, N. (2004) An absence of evidence linking perceived memory problems to the menopause. *British Journal of General Practice*, 54(503), 434–38.

Freedman, R.R. (2005) Pathophysiology and treatment of menopausal hot flushes. *Seminars in Reproductive Medicine*, 23(2), 117–25.

Freedman, R.R. and Woodward, S. (1992) Behavioral treatment of menopausal hot flushes: evaluation by ambulatory monitoring. *American Journal Obstetrics Gynecology*, 167(2), 436–39.

Freeman, E.W. and Sherif, K. (2007) Prevalence of hot flushes and night sweats around the world: a systematic review. *Climacteric*, 10(3), 197–214.

Freeman, E.W., Sammel, M.D. and Richard, J. (2014) Risk of long-term hot flushes after natural menopause: evidence from the Penn Ovarian Aging Study cohort. *Menopause*. DOI: 10.1097/GME.0000000000000196.

Gannon, L., Hansel, S. and Goodwin, J. (1987) Correlates of menopausal hot flushes. *Journal of Behavioural Medicine*, 10(3), 277–85.

Germaine, L.M. and Freedman, R.R. (1984) Behavioural treatment of menopausal hot flushes: Evaluation by objective methods. *Journal of Consulting Clinical Psychology*, 1(52), 1072–79.

Gold, E.B., Colvin, A., Avis, N., Bromberger, J., Greendale, G.A., Powell, L. et al. (2006) Longitudinal analysis of the association between vasomotor symptoms and race/ethnicity across the menopausal transition: Study of Women's Health Across the Nation. *American Journal Public Health*, 96(7), 1226–35.

Greene, J.G. (1998) Constructing a standard climacteric scale. *Maturitas*, 61(1), 78–84.

Gupta, P., Sturdee, D.W. and Hunter, M.S. (2006a) Mid-aged health in women from the Indian subcontinent (MAHWIS): general health and the experience of the menopause in women. *Climacteric*, 9(1), 13–22.

Gupta, P., Sturdee, D.W., Palin, S., Majumder, K., Fear, R., Marshall, T. et al. (2006b) Menopausal symptoms in women treated for breast cancer: the prevalence and severity of symptoms and their perceived effects on quality of life. *Climacteric*, 9(1), 49–58.

Guthrie, J.R., Dennerstein, L., Taffe, J.R. and Donnelly, V. (2003) Health care seeking for menopausal problems. *Climacteric*, 6(2), 112–17.

Harlow, S.D., Gass, M., Hall, J.E., Lobo, R., Maki, P., Rebar, R.W. et al (2012) Executive summary of the Stages of Reproductive Ageing Workshop +10: addressing the unfinished agenda of staging reproductive aging. *Menopause*, 19(4), 105–14.

Harvey, A.G. (2002) A cognitive model of insomnia. *Behaviour Research and Therapy*, 40(8), 869–93.

Hayes, S.C., Follette, V.M. and Lineham, M.M. (2004) *Mindfulness and acceptance: expanding the cognitive behavioural tradition*. New York: Guildford.

Henderson, V.W. (2009) Menopause, cognitive aging and dementia: practice implications. *Menopause International*, 15(1), 41–44.

Hersh, A., Stefanick, M. and Stafford, R. (2004) National use of postmenopausal hormone therapy: annual trends and response to recent evidence. *Journal of the American Medical Association*, 291(1), 47–53.

Hershman, D.L., Shao, T., Kushi, L.H. et al. (2011) Early discontinuation and non-adherence to adjuvant hormonal therapy are associated with increased mortality in women with breast cancer. *Breast Cancer Research and Treatment*, 126(2), 529–37.

Howell, A., Cuzick, J., Baum, M., Buzdar, A., Dowsett, M., Forbes, J.F. et al. (2005) Results of the ATAC (Arimidex, Tamoxifen, Alone or in Combination) trial after completion of 5 years' adjuvant treatment for breast cancer. *The Lancet*, 365(9453), 60–62.

Hunter, M.S. (1992) The Women's Health Questionnaire: a measure of mid-aged women's perceptions of their emotional and physical health. *Psychology and Health*, 7(1), 45–54.

Hunter, M.S. (2003) Cognitive behavioural interventions for premenstrual and menopausal problems. *Journal of Reproductive Infant Psychology*, 21(3), 183–94.

Hunter, M.S. and Chilcot, J. (2013) Testing a cognitive model of menopausal hot flushes and night sweats. *Journal of Psychosomatic Research*, 74(4), 307–12.

Hunter, M.S. and Liao, K.L.M. (1995) A psychological analysis of menopausal hot flushes. *British Journal of Clinical Psychology*, 34(4), 589–99.

Hunter, M.S. and Liao, K.L.M. (1996) Evaluation of a four-session cognitive-behavioural intervention for menopausal hot flushes. *British Journal of Health Psychology*, 1(2), 113–25.

Hunter, M.S. and Mann, E. (2010) A cognitive model of menopausal hot flushes. *Journal of Psychosomatic Research*, 69, 491–501.

Hunter, M.S. and O'Dea, I. (1997) Menopause: Bodily changes and multiple meanings, in J.M. Ussher (ed.) *Body talk: the material and discursive regulation of sexuality, madness and reproduction*. London: Routledge, pp. 199–222.

Hunter, M.S. and O'Dea, I. (2001) Cognitive appraisal of the menopause: the menopause representations questionnaire (MRQ). *Psychology, Health and Medicine*, 6(1), 65–76.

Hunter, M.S. and Rendall, M. (2007) Bio-psycho–socio-cultural perspectives on menopause. *Best Practice and Research Clinical Obstetrics & Gynaecology*, 21(2), 261–74.

Hunter, M.S. and Smith, M. (2013) *Managing hot flushes and night sweats: a cognitive behavioural self-help guide to the menopause*. Sussex, UK: Routledge.

Hunter, M.S., Ayers, B. and Smith, M. (2011) The Hot Flush Behaviour Scale: a measure of behavioural reactions to menopausal hot flushes and night sweats. *Menopause*, 18(11), 1178–83.

Hunter, M.S., O'Dea, I. and Britten, N. (1997) Decision-making and hormone replacement therapy: a qualitative study. *Social Science Medicine*, 45(10), 1541–48.

Hunter, M.S., Coventry, S., Mendes, N. and Grunfeld, E.A. (2009a) Evaluation of a group cognitive behavioural intervention for women suffering from menopausal symptoms following breast cancer treatment. *Psycho-Oncology*, 18(5), 560–63.

Hunter, M.S., Coventry, S., Mendes, N. and Grunfeld, E.A. (2009b) Menopausal symptoms following breast cancer treatment: a qualitative investigation of cognitive and behavioural responses. *Maturitas*, 63(4), 336–40.

Hunter, M.S., Grunfeld, E.A., Mittal, S., Sikka, P., Ramirez, A.J. and Fentiman, I. (2004) Menopausal symptoms in women with breast cancer: prevalence and treatment preferences. *Psycho-Oncology*, 13(11), 769–78.

Hunter, M.S., Gentry-Maharaj, A., Ryan, A., Burnell, M., Lanceley, A., Fraser, L. et al. (2012) Prevalence, frequency and problem-rating of hot flushes persist in older postmenopausal women: impact of age, BMI, hysterectomy, lifestyle and mood in a cross sectional cohort study of 10,418 British women aged 54–65. *British Journal of Obstetrics and Gynaecology*, 119(1), 40–50.

Hvas, L. (2006) Menopausal women's positive experience of growing older. *Maturitas*, 54(3), 245–51.

Innes, K.E., Selfe, T.K. and Vishnu, A. (2010) Mind–body therapies for menopausal symptoms: a systematic review. *Maturitas*, 66(2), 135–49.

Irvin, J.H., Domar, A.D., Clark, C., Zuttermeister, P.C. et al. (1996) The effects of relaxation response training on menopausal symptoms. *Journal of Psychosomatic Obstetrics and Gynaecology*, 17(4), 202–207.

Irwin, M.R., Cole, J.C. and Nicassio, P.M. (2006) Comparative meta-analysis of behavioural interventions for insomnia and their efficacy in middle-aged adults and in older adults 55+ years of age. *Health Psychology*, 25(1), 3–14.

Kabat-Zinn, J. (2003) Mindfulness-based interventions in context: past, present, and future. *Clinical Psychology: Science and Practice*, 10(2), 144–56.

Kadakia, K.C., Loprinzi, C.L. and Barton, D.L. (2012) Hot flushes: the ongoing search for effective interventions. *Menopause*, 19(7), 719–21.

Keefer, L. and Blanchard, E.B. (2005) A behavioural group treatment program for menopausal hot flushes. *Applied Psychophysiology and Biofeedback*, 30(1), 21–30.

Leventhal, H., Nerenz, D. and Steel, D.J. (1984) Illness representations and coping with health threats. In Baum, A., Taylor, S.E. and Singer, J.E. (eds) *Handbook of Psychology and Health*. Erlbaum: Illsdale, pp. 126–42.

Lock, M. (2005) Cross-cultural vasomotor symptoms reporting: conceptual and methodological issues. *Menopause*, 12(3), 239–41.

Mann, E., Smith, M.J., Balabanovic, J., Hellier, J., Hamed, H., Grunfeld, B. and Hunter, M.S. (2012) Efficacy of a cognitive behavioural intervention to treat menopausal symptoms following breast cancer treatment (MENOS 1): a randomised controlled trial. *Lancet Oncology*, 13(3), 309–18.

Marques, E.A., Mota, J. and Carvalho, J. (2012) Exercise effects on bone mineral density in older adults: a meta-analysis of randomized controlled trials. *Age*, 34(6), 1493–515.

Melby, M.K., Lock, M. and Kaufert, P. (2005) Culture and symptom reporting at menopause. *Human Reproductive Update*, 11(5), 495–512.

Menon, U., Burnell, M., Sharma, A., Gentry-Maharaj, A., Fraser, L., Parmar, M. et al. (2007) Decline in use of hormone therapy among postmenopausal women in the United Kingdom. *Menopause*, 14(3), 462–67.

Mishra, G.D. and Kuh, D. (2012) Health symptoms during midlife in relation to menopausal transition: British prospective cohort study. *British Medical Journal*, 344, e402.

Mitchell, E.S. and Woods, N.F. (2011) Cognitive symptoms during the menopausal transition and early postmenopause. *Climacteric*, 14(2), 252–61.

Morgan, A. and Fenlon, D. on behalf of the NCRI CSG Breast Cancer Working Party on Symptom Management. (2014) Is it me or is it hot in here – a plea for more research into hot flushes. *Journal of Clinical Oncology* (in press).

Nelson, H.D., Vesco, K.K., Haney, E., Fu, R., Nedrow, A., Miller, J. et al. (2006) Non-hormonal therapies for menopausal hot flushes. *Journal of the American Medical Association*, 295(17), 2057–71.

Norton, S., Chilcot, J. and Hunter, M.S. (2014) Cognitive behaviour therapy for menopausal symptoms (hot flushes and night sweats): moderators and mediators of treatment effects. *Menopause*, 21(6), 574–78.

Panay, N. and Fenton, A. (2008) Premature ovarian failure: a growing concern. *Climacteric*, 11(1), 1–3.

Pennebaker, J.W. (1982) *The psychology of physical symptoms*. New York: Springer.

Perz, J. and Ussher, J.M. (2008) 'The horror of this living decay': women's negotiation and resistance of medical discourses around menopause and midlife. *Women's Studies International Forum*, 31(4), 293–99.

Pitkin, J. (2012) Alternative and complementary therapies for the menopause. *Menopause International*, 18(1), 20–27.

Rada, G., Capurro, D., Pantoja, T., Corbalán, J., Moreno, G., Letelier, L.M. et al. (2010) Non-hormonal interventions for hot flushes in women with a history of breast cancer. *The Cochrane Library*, issue 9.

Rendall, M.J., Simonds, L.M. and Hunter, M.S. (2008) The Hot Flush Beliefs Scale: a tool for assessing thoughts and beliefs associated with the experience of menopausal hot flushes and night sweats. *Maturitas*, 60(2), 158–69.

Reynolds, F. (1999) Some relationships between perceived control and women's reported coping strategies for menopausal hot flushes. *Maturitas*, 32(1), 25–32.

Reynolds, F. (2000) Relationships between catastrophic thoughts, perceived control and distress during menopausal hot flushes: exploring the correlates of a questionnaire measure. *Maturitas*, 36(2), 113–22.

Richardson, S. (1993) The biological basis of the menopause. In Burger, H.G. (ed.) *The Menopause: Clinical Endocrinology and Metabolism*. London: Balliere Tindall, pp. 1–16.

Rossouw, J.E., Anderson, G.L., Prentice, R.L., LaCroix, A.Z., Kooperberg, C., Stefanick, M.L. et al. (2002) Risks and benefits of oestrogen plus progestin in healthy postmenopausal women: Principal results from the Women's Health Initiative randomized controlled trial. *Journal of the American Medical Association*, 288(3), 321–33.

Schierbeck, L.L., Rejnmark, L., Tofteng, C.L., Eiken, P., Mosekilde, L., Kober, L. et al. (2012) Effect of hormone replacement therapy on cardiovascular events in recently postmenopausal women: randomised trial. *British Medical Journal*, 345, 6409.

Sherman, S. (2005) Defining the menopausal transition. *The American Journal of Medicine*, 118(12S), 3–7.

Sievert, L.L., Obermayer, C.M. and Price, K. (2006) Determinants of hot flushes and night sweats. *Annals Human Biology*, 33, 4–16.

Smith, M.J., Mann, E., Mirza, A. and Hunter, M.S. (2011) Men and women's perceptions of hot flushes within social situations: are menopausal women's negative beliefs valid? *Maturitas*, 69, 57–62.

Sprague, B.L., Trentham-Dietz, A. and Cronin, K.A.A. (2012) Sustained decline in postmenopausal hormone use: results from the National Health and Nutrition Examination Survey, 1999–2010. *Obstetrics & Gynecology*, 120(3), 595–603.

Stefanopoulou, E. and Hunter, M.S. (2013) Does pattern recognition software using the Bahr monitor improve sensitivity, specificity and concordance of ambulatory skin conductance monitoring of hot flushes. *Menopause*, 20(11), 1133–38.

Stevenson, D.W. and Delprato, D.J. (1983) Multiple component self-control programme for menopausal hot flushes. *Journal of Behaviour Therapy and Experimental Psychiatry*, 14(2), 137–40.

Suvanto-Luukkonen, E., Koivunen, R., Sundstrom, H., Bloigu, R., Karjalainen, E., Haiva-Mallinen, L. et al. (2005) Citalopram and fluoxetine in the treatment of postmenopausal symptoms: a prospective, randomized 9 month placebo controlled double blind study. *Menopause*, 12(1), 18–26.

Swartzman, L.C., Edelberg, R. and Kemmann, E. (1990) Impact of stress on objectively recorded menopausal hot flushes and on flush report bias. *Health Psychology*, 9(5), 529–45.

Thewes, B., Butow, P., Girgis, A. and Pendlebury, S. (2004) The psychosocial needs of breast cancer survivors: a qualitative study of the shared and unique needs of younger versus older survivors. *Psycho-Oncology*, 13(3), 3177–89.

Thurston, R.C., Sowers, M.R., Sutton-Tyrrell, K., Everson-Rose, S.A., Lewis, T.T., Edmundowicz, D. et al. (2008) Abdominal adiposity and hot flushes among midlife women. *Menopause*, 15(3), 429–34.

Thurston, R.C., Sowers, M.F.R., Sternfeld, B., Gold, E.B., Bromberger, J., Chang, Y. et al. (2009) Gains in body fat and vasomotor symptom reporting over the menopausal transition. The study of women's health across the nation. *American Journal of Epidemiology*, 170(6), 766–74.

Tremblay, A., Sheeran, L. and Aranda, S.K. (2008) Psychoeducational interventions to alleviate hot flushes: a systematic review. *Menopause*, 15(1), 193–202.

Ussher, J.M., Perz, J., Gilbert, E., Wong, W.K.T. and Hobbs, K. (2013) Renegotiating sex and intimacy after cancer: resisting the coital imperative. *Cancer Nursing*, 36(6), 454–62.

Utian, W. (2005) Psychosocial and socioeconomic burden of vasomotor symptoms in menopause: a comprehensive review. *Health and Quality of Life Outcomes*, 3(1), 47–57.

Wijma, K., Melin, A., Nedstrand, E. and Hammar, M. (1997) Treatment of menopausal symptoms with applied relaxation: a pilot study. *Journal of Behaviour and Experimental Psychiatry*, 28(4), 251–61.

Wilbush, J. (1979) La Menespausie – the birth of a syndrome. *Maturitas*, 1, 145–51.

Winterich, J.A. (2003) Sex, menopause and culture: sexual orientation and the meaning of menopause for women's sex lives. *Gender and Society*, 17(4), 627–42.

Woods, N.F., Mariella, A. and Mitchell, E.S. (2006) Depressed mood symptoms during the menopausal transition: observations from the Seattle Midlife Women's Health study. *Climacteric*, 9(3), 195–203.

World Health Organization. (1981) *Research on Menopause. Report of a WHO Scientific group*. WHO technical report N670. WHO Geneva.

Index

acceptance 15, 35
aches and pains 2 *see also* pain
adrenal glands 3
age: negative attitudes 2–4, 7, 23, 46–7, 90–3
agenda: session one 21; session two 30; session three 44; session four 60; session five 74; session six 84
alcohol 6, 9, 31, 67, 94
alternative therapies 10
anger 20, 53–5, 87
anti-depressants *see* SSRIs
anxiety 2, 50–1, 59; behaviour 7, 9, 15, 31, 56; evolutionary roots 33; group participants 17, 20; hot flushes 5, 6, 8, 48–9; sleep 76, 80; thinking 7, 48, 77
assumptions *see* cognitive biases
Athena Network 182
attitudes to menopause 3–4, 90–1 *see also* menopause: beliefs
attentional focus 75
avoidance *see* anxiety; behaviour

behavioural activation *see* pleasant activities
behavioural experiment 9, 71
black cohosh 10
body fat distribution 93
body focus *see* somatic amplification
body image 93–4
body mass index 5 *see also* weight
breast cancer 22, 82, 89–90; emotional responses 23, 29; fatigue 69–70; hot flushes 1, 5, 54–5; HRT 10; sleep 64
Breast Cancer Campaign 178
Breast Cancer Care 177
British Association for Behavioural and Cognitive Psychotherapy 180
British Menopause Society 175
British Psychological Society 179

caffeine 6, 19, 25, 31, 62, 67
Cancer Research UK 178
Careline 181
Carers UK 181
chemotherapy 5
children 2, 29
classical conditioning 68
Clonidine 10
Coffee *see* caffeine
cognition *see* thinking
cognitive biases 50; catastrophising 49, 52, 78; mind reading 50; observer perspective 50; 'shoulds' 52; sleep related 71
cognitive restructuring 35–7, 49–50, 55–6, 75, 78–81; complexity of 60, 74; continuum work 77–8
complementary therapies *see* alternative therapies
concentration 2, 65, 94
confidentiality 16, 20–1
control 7, 12, 52–3, 55, 59
cooling behaviours 7, 15, 31, 48–9, 56
cross cultural differences 2–3
Cruse Bereavement Service 181

Daisy Network 176
dementia 16, 25–6
depression 2, 38–9, 46, 85, 179–80; primary care treatment 13
Depression Alliance 180
diaphragmatic breathing *see* paced breathing
diet 67, 93, 94
Divorce Support Group 182
dizziness 52–4
dry skin 2

early menopause 1, 5, 10, 16, 53, 82, 91, 94
e-book 16
elderly relatives 2, 29
embarrassment 50
ending intervention 95–6
energy *see* fatigue
evening primrose oil 10
exercise 5,12, 29, 35, 38, 67, 71, 93–5

fatigue 2, 29, 31, 62, 64, 71, 78 *see also* breast cancer: fatigue
femininity 46
Fertility Friends 176
fight or flight response *see* anxiety
follicle stimulating hormone 2–3
frustration 52–4, 76–7

Gapapentin 10
General practitioner 13, 84, 94
goal setting 22–3, 31, 40, 43, 59, 71–4, 80, 87–8
grandchildren 29
Greene Climacteric Scale 15

group CBT: assessment for 13–16; attendance 19, 21; exclusion criteria 13; expectations 20–2; good-byes and debrief 95–6; ground rules 16–17, 19; introductions 19; outside pressures 74; planning 17–18; rationale 10–13, 15
group support 37

health anxiety 29
herbal remedies 10
high standards 50
homework 12, 19, 28–31, 42–6, 59, 72–4, 76, 84–6
hopelessness 20
hormone replacement therapy, hormone therapy *see* HRT
Hot Flush Behaviour Scale 15
Hot Flush Belief Scale 14
Hot Flush Diary 14–15, 57, 96
Hot Flush Rating Scale 11, 13–14, 96
hot flushes: 4–5; behaviours 51, 55–6, 81 see also cooling behaviours; causes 5–6 *see also* thermo neutral zone; cognitive behavioural model 8–10, 19, 24–5, 47–8, 50, 73, 80–1; frequency 9, 13; negative consequences 4,7; personal accounts 50, 54, 61, 75; prevalence 7; psychological factors 6–9, 11, 43–4, 47–50, 54, 56, 60–1, 72–4, 81
HRT 1, 5, 10, 94
hypothalamo-pituitary-ovarian axis 3
hypothalamus 5
hysterectomy 2

Increasing Access to Psychological Therapy (IAPT) Service 178
insomnia 2; anxiety 62, 64, 66; behaviours 70; cognitive behavioural model 59, 71, 73; daytime tiredness 62, 64, 66–7, 71; thinking *see also* sleep
International Menopause Society 175
irritability 2, 52

job *see* work
joint pain *see* pain

libido 2, 92–3 *see also* sexual functioning
life events 2, 4
lifestyle 3, 31
loss of energy *see* fatigue

Macmillan Cancer Support 178
maintaining changes 83–8
maintenance plan *see* maintaining changes
managing pain *see* pain
memory 2, 12, 65, 82, 94
menopause: adjustment across menopause transition 90–1; beliefs 3–4, 7, 9, 11, 23–4, 43, 46–8; definitions and stages 1–2; other people's views 51; personal accounts 22; positive consequences 17, 74; socio-cultural influences 2–3 *see also* early menopause
Menopause Exchange 176
Menopause Matters 176
Menopause Support 176
MENOS studies 11–12
menstrual cycle 1–2
Mind 179
mood: menopause 3–4; sleep 71; swings 2; *see also* depression
Moodjuice 179
motivation 53, 87, 93, 96

napping 62, 68–9
NHS Live Well 177
National Institute of Clinical Excellence: menopause guidelines 10
National Osteoporosis Society 94, 178
nausea 52–54
nicotine 67
night sweats 59, 62, 65, 70, 73, 75–6, 79–80; routine response 80 *see also* sleep
night time waking 63 see also insomnia
non-hormonal treatments 10
No Panic 180
nor epinephrine 6
North American Menopause Society 175
Northumberland, Tyne and Wear NHS Foundation Trust 179

oestrogen 3, 5, 23
oopherectomy 2
open discussion 88–95
osteoporosis 82, 94
ovaries 2–3

paced breathing 9–12, 13, 15, 26–8, 41–3, 53–4, 56, 59–61, 70, 73–6, 79–80, 83, 87
pacing 29, 35, 39, 71, 95
pain 83, 95
panic 52
pleasant activities 29, 35, 38–9
positive psychology 35, 37
precipitants *see* triggers
premature menopause *see* early menopause
problem solving 29, 35, 39–40, 79
progressive muscle relaxation 26–7, 41
psychoeducation 9–10, 19; hot flushes 23–5; sleep 59, 63, 77–8; stress 32–3; thinking 52–3

references 183–8
Relate 181
relationships 2, 29, 31
relaxation 9–11, 19–20, 26–9, 40–3, 56, 59, 67, 69–70, 71–6, 79, 80, 95
resources 96, 175–82
review 83–8
role change 2
role play 61, 73, 75
Royal College of Psychiatrists 179

Samaritans 180
selective serotonin reuptake inhibitors *see* SSRIs
self criticism 35–7, 49–50
self efficacy 9
self help CBT intervention 16
self help study *see* MENOS studies
self image 50, 77 *see also* body image
self regulation theory 8
serotonin 6
setbacks 87
sexual functioning 4, 68, 82, 92–3 *see also* libido
shame 50
skin conductance 9, 12
sleep 7, 73, 76; behaviours 7, 62, 73, 79; beliefs 64–5, 77, 79–80; CBT model 7, 9, 66; diary 43, 57, 59, 62–3; environment 67–8, 76; perceptions 65–6, 76, 78; quantity 62, 64, 76–7; stages 63, 78; *see also* insomnia
sleep hygiene 59, 67, 75
sleep scheduling 59, 67, 70, 76
smoking 5, 9, 94
social anxiety: hot flushes 7, 50–2
social situations 43, 51–2, 59
somatic amplification 9, 50, 53
SSRIs 10
Stages of Reproductive Ageing Workshop (STRAW) 2, *see also* menopause: definitions and stages
stimulus control 67–70
stress 3–4, 6, 8–9, 24, 26, 29, 76–7, 79, 81, 93; cognitive behavioural approach 33–5, 42, 74, 77; management 29–32, 35–40, 43, 48–50, 56, 59–60, 72–4, 79–81; personal examples 44–6
summarising intervention 87
supervision 1, 17
surgical menopause 1, 4–5, 16
symptom perception theory 8

Tamoxifen 5, 12
Testosterone 3
thermo-neutral zone 5–6, 19, 23–4, 30–1, 81 *see also* hot flushes
thinking: anxious 7, 33–5, 78 *see also* cognitive biases; behaviour 35, 50 *see also* cognitive biases *and* cognitive restructuring
tiredness *see* fatigue
training 1,17–18,
transition 2
triggers 6, 9, 19, 25–6, 30–1, 42–3, 59–60, 81
Turn2me 180

uncertainty 23

vaginal dryness 2, 4, 92
vasomotor symptoms *see* hot flushes
vitamins 10

weight 82, 93–4 *see also* body mass index
wild yam 10
wind down routine 67, 69, 76
Women's Health 177
Women's Health Concern 177
Women's Health London 177
Women's Health Questionnaire 15
World Health Organization 1 *see also* menopause definitions and stages
work 29, 33–4, 36–7, 45, 51, 54, 74, 76–8, 86, 89–92
worry 66, 69, 73, 76, 79